ESSENTIAL
ARMS

D0406694

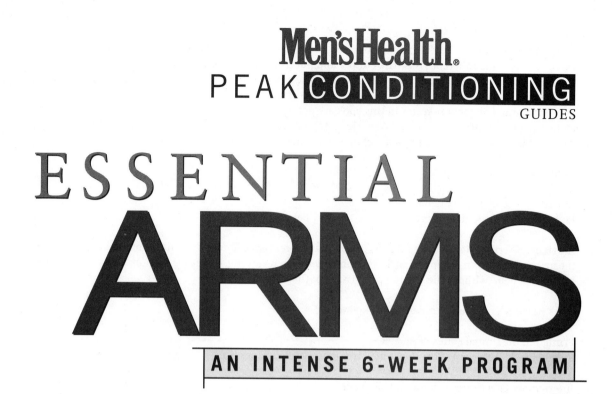

Men's Health®
PEAK CONDITIONING GUIDES

ESSENTIAL
ARMS

AN INTENSE 6-WEEK PROGRAM

BY
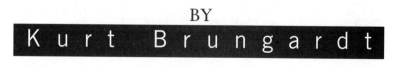
Kurt Brungardt

RODALE®

Notice

The information in this book is meant to supplement, not replace, proper exercise training. All forms of exercise pose some inherent risks. The editors and publisher advise readers to take full responsibility for their safety and know their limits. Before practicing the exercises in this book, be sure that your equipment is well-maintained, and do not take risks beyond your level of experience, aptitude, training, and fitness. The exercise and dietary programs in this book are not intended as a substitute for any exercise routine or dietary regimen that may have been prescribed by your doctor. As with all exercise and dietary programs, you should get your doctor's approval before beginning.

© 2001 by Kurt Brungardt

Illustrations © by Karen Kuchar
Photographs © by Rodale Inc., except page 14, © by Bettman/CORBIS

All rights reserved. No part of this publication may be reproduced or transmitted in any form or by any means, electronic or mechanical, including photocopying, recording, or any other information storage and retrieval system, without the written permission of the publisher.

Men's Health is a registered trademark of Rodale Inc.

Printed in the United States of America
Rodale Inc. makes every effort to use acid-free ∞, recycled paper ♻

Interior and Cover Designer: Susan P. Eugster
Interior and Cover Photographer: Mitch Mandel/Rodale Images

Library of Congress Cataloging-in-Publication Data

Brungardt, Kurt, 1964-
    Essential arms : an intense 6-week program / by Kurt Brungardt.
        p.   cm. — (Men's health peak conditioning guides)
    Includes index.
    ISBN 1-57954-308-1 paperback
    1. Exercise. 2. Arm exercises. I. Title. II. Series.
    GV5Q8 .B793 2001
    613.7'13—dc21   2001002149

Distributed to the book trade by St. Martin's Press

   4 6 8 10 9 7 5 3   paperback

Visit us on the Web at www.menshealthbooks.com, or call us toll-free at (800) 848-4735.

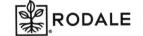

RODALE

WE **INSPIRE** AND **ENABLE** PEOPLE TO IMPROVE
THEIR LIVES AND THE WORLD AROUND THEM

CONTENTS

INTRODUCTION

I grew up in a small world. Everyone lived in smaller houses than people prefer nowadays, our parents drove station wagons instead of minivans and SUVs, and the people themselves were relative shrimps.

Almost nobody lifted weights. Okay, maybe the high school quarterback had dumbbells in his garage. Everyone else pretty much went through life with the muscles that his genetics, lifestyle, and job offered him. At my school, the hard-working janitor had the biggest muscles. The deskbound principal, I would guess, had the smallest. (I have to hedge my memories on the principal's physique because, to my knowledge, no one ever saw the man in anything but a suit and tie.)

I started lifting weights at a very early age—13, I believe. By the time I graduated from high school in 1975, I had a total of a half-dozen schoolmates who shared my passion for pumping iron. We didn't know squat about lifting, and only one of us got results that were noticeable on first glance. (He was promptly nicknamed Herk, short for Hercules.) I could see the minor differences that I had created in my own developing body, but I'm pretty sure I was the only one who could. My arms were still so skinny that I could roll up my sleeves all the way to the shoulder seams without meeting any resistance.

The hulkification of America began the following year, when Sylvester Stallone removed his shirt for Talia Shire in *Rocky*. In the minds of millions of adolescent males, boxer Rocky Balboa's quest for self-respect was forever linked with his impressive biceps development.

Pumping Iron hit theaters a year later, featuring Arnold Schwarzenegger's famous comment that the pump you get from lifting is better than an orgasm.

Couple the aftereffects of those two movies with a parallel rise in the Jane Fonda culture, and exercise became an integral part of life for a significant minority of Americans. Men saw bigger muscles as a ticket to better sexual opportunity, improved sports performance, and—perhaps most important—the envy of other men.

Unfortunately, despite our desire to get bigger and stronger, we still didn't know the best ways to build muscle. I didn't really learn how to get the results I wanted until the late 1990s—almost 30 years after I started lifting. That's when I finally figured out how to manipulate workouts and meals to get the maximum benefit from the effort I was willing and able to expend. (By then, I had a wife, three children, and a mortgage—a nice life, but a hell of a set of obstacles to overcome when trying to find time to exercise.)

The author of this book, Kurt Brungardt, figured all this out a lot sooner than I did. The first book in his midsection trilogy, *The Complete Book of Abs*, created the abdominal-exercise genre when it was published in 1993 and remains one of its bestsellers. His *Men of Steel: Abs of Steel* remains one of the few exercise videos that males have ever felt compelled to buy.

This the second book by Kurt in the *Men's Health* Peak Conditioning Guides series. The first, *Essential Abs*, served as an introduction to exercise in general as well as an indispensable guide to flattening and shaping a supersize belly.

The emphasis here shifts to pure muscle-building. Kurt assumes that a guy who wants bigger arms is prepared to step into the weight room to put in some serious sweat equity. But this is still a beginner-friendly book that walks you through the basics of exercise at the same time that it gently nudges you toward more advanced arm-building exercises and techniques. Moreover, it's the perfect manual for an expanding world. It helps you upsize the parts of your body that seem too small by modern standards, while keeping the rest of your physique under control.

I wish I'd had this book back in 1970, when I picked up my first barbell. Having bigger muscles in my formative years sure would've made those years a lot more interesting. But it's also nice to know that, thanks to Kurt, you can condense my 30-year learning curve into the 6-week Core Program that's the heart of *Essential Arms*.

I'll see you in the weight room. You'll know me because I'll be throwing off the intense older-but-wiser vibe. I'll know you because, thanks to this book, you'll look like you know what you're doing.

—Lou Schuler
FITNESS DIRECTOR
MEN'S HEALTH MAGAZINE

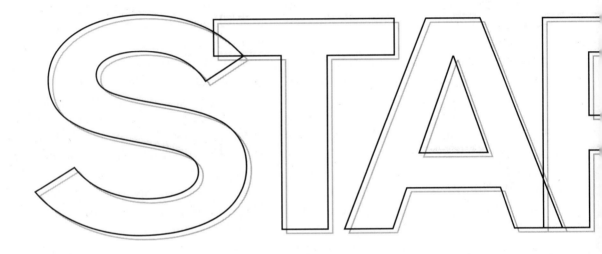

PART ONE

RTING
UP

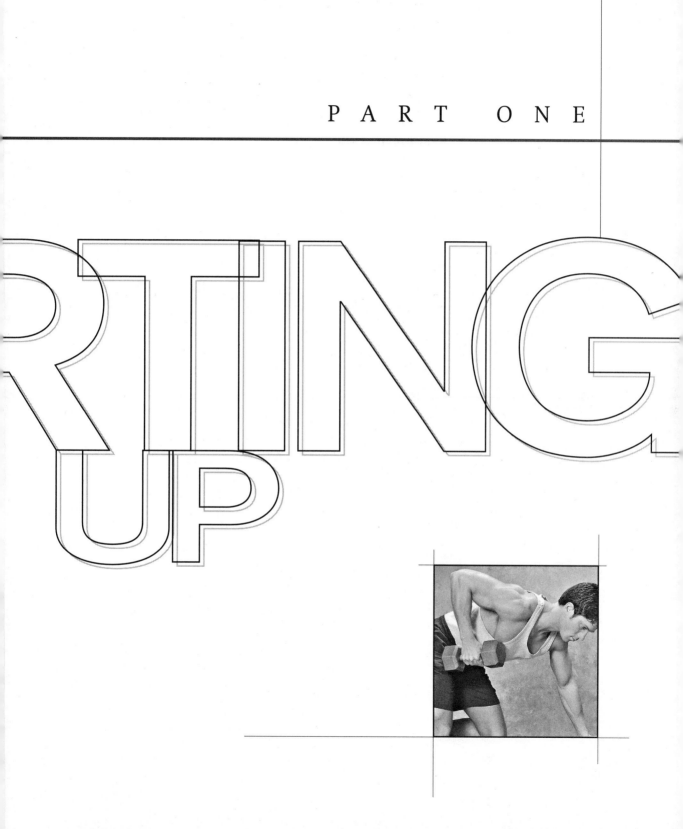

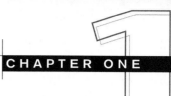

CHAPTER ONE

ESSENTIAL
ARMS PLAN

It's not a rational goal. It won't help us get rich or live longer or save the world. And yet we want it, and we'll spend almost any amount of time pursuing it. The quest for powerful arms—Himalayan biceps and ox-bow triceps and forearms like jumbo bags of Twizzlers—is illogical but compelling nonetheless.

This book will give you a definitive system to put you on target for bigger guns. It will explain the basics of building muscle and launch you into the Core Program, a 6-week routine featuring the best arm exercises for beginners. It will walk you through the best dietary strategy for maximizing muscle and minimizing fat. It will give you a solid total-body strength-training program and help you understand why it's important to build all your muscles even if your immediate goal is just bigger arms. Finally, it will provide six advanced arm-building routines that will work your arm muscles in a slightly different way, meaning you'll continue to get bigger, stronger arms long after you've finished the 6-week Core Program.

THE INTENDED READER

By now, you've probably figured out that this book isn't for the guy whose résumé will one day include professional wrestling. It addresses the needs of guys who are tired of walking around with weak, underdeveloped *Tyrannosaurus rex* arms. These guys will see the biggest gains, though it will take them the longest.

Essential Arms is also for very fit guys—athletes, even—who've never begun a formal program aimed at upsizing their arms. With their base of fitness, these guys will probably get fast results on the Core Program and see sensational gains when they try the advanced programs in chapter 13.

Finally, this book takes into consideration confused guys who've been hitting the gym but who've never found a system they could stick with long enough to truly change the size and appearance of their arms. The Core Program will show them the benefits of sticking with one program for 6 weeks, and it'll clarify what's been going wrong in all those months or years of fruitless exercise.

WHAT'S INSIDE

Whatever your fitness level, here's what *Essential Arms* has for you.

- Basic arm-muscle anatomy
- A stretching routine that keeps you limber from head to toe
- Proper technique for the most effective arm-building exercises
- A total-body exercise routine that harnesses the power of your body's most powerful muscle-building hormones
- A progressive week-by-week program
- Nutritional know-how to ensure that your sweat and effort result in bigger muscles, not just tired ones
- Advanced arm-enlarging routines

This book is broken down into four basic parts. Part one will teach you the truth about building muscle in general and arm muscles in particular. Part two will teach you principles and techniques for safe and effective arm training. Part three will guide you through the Core Program of fundamental arm exercises. Finally, part four will show you advanced routines and make sure you understand how to keep building and maintaining muscle for the rest of your life.

ESSENTIAL CONSISTENCY

Until human physiology changes, the basics of building muscle will remain the same. So whether you've snapped up this book hot off the presses in the year 2001 or dusted it off in your grandfather's attic in 2061, the exercises it offers should be just as effective for you.

But you won't get the full message of this book unless you keep reading, every page, right to the end. You can't stop in the middle and expect to know everything you need to know about muscular arms. The exercises inside work the same way—if you want to get the complete physical benefits, you have to keep doing them, every workout, without giving up. Your bulging biceps and rippling triceps will come from high-quality exercise, done consistently. Individual bodies progress at different speeds, but no matter what your genetics, consistency is the key to progress.

Gentlemen, flex those biceps—it's time to build some muscle.

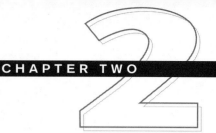

CHAPTER TWO

ESSENTIAL
FACTS

Since you're a man, you're probably not parading around in shirts that end 2 inches above your trousers and trousers that start 2 inches below your navel. So your rippling abdominal muscles remain hidden from the world at large. Nor are you wearing scoop-top shirts to expose your swollen pectorals. And, if you spend most of your days in an office, your pants hide your fantastically muscled legs, and your shirt keeps your broad-as-a-six-lane-highway deltoids under wraps.

In fact, there's only one muscle group you're allowed to expose on a daily basis: your arms. But while we'd all prefer to have Arnold Schwarzenegger–size appendages protruding from the sleeves of our sport shirts on casual Friday, a lot of us would have trouble outflexing Maria Shriver.

No problem. We all have to start somewhere—even Arnold was a skinny little kid at one point (when he was 6, maybe). However, before you start fantasizing about turning the last page of this book with arms like the Terminator's, here's a word from our sponsor: reality.

THE TRUTH ABOUT ARMATURE

If you look at pictures of circus strongmen and body-builders from the late 19th and early 20th centuries (including "The World's Most Perfectly Developed Man,"

Charles Atlas, shown at left), you see sculpted midsections, wide shoulders, muscular chests and backs, thick and athletic legs . . . and, by today's standards, relatively skinny arms.

So what changed between then and now? The development of anabolic steroids. The reason that so many men today have arms like well-fed pythons is because they've had some injectable assistance.

It's certainly possible to build fantastic-looking arms with smart exercise and good nutrition—we're going to show you how to do it. But you can't expect to get arms like Arnold's, because Arnold used steroids. He also trained hard and had genetically magnificent biceps structure. Still, he wouldn't have grown to the proportions he did without the help of steroids.

Same goes for the professional body-builders you see on magazines and many of the athletes you watch on *Monday Night Football* and in the Olympics, World Series, and NBA finals. If a guy's arms are considerably bigger than the arms of athletes, models, and musclemen from the pre-steroid era (in other words, before the early 1960s), you can bet your paycheck that either he's on the juice or he has juiced in the past. Steroids permanently change muscle architecture, particularly in the arms, shoulders, chest, and upper back. So a guy who 'roided for a few years and then quit can still grow bigger, thicker, more impressive muscles than a guy who never has.

This is the last time this book will mention steroids. They don't have anything to do with you. Just remember this: The biggest arms you see in magazines, movies, and sports competitions are about as natural as most of the breasts you see in magazines, movies, and sports competitions (on the cheerleaders, of course). If you don't want to take steroids—and if you really want to be fit and healthy, you don't—you can't expect to build arms that look like those.

MYTHS AND FACTS

Despite the fact that men spend a disproportionate amount of time training their arms, they rarely see the fruits of that labor. This is due to fundamental mistakes in their arm training. Let's clear up some of the misinformation that hinders the average guy.

Myth: If I want big arms, I have to dedicate one or two workouts a week to arm exercises.

Fact: Workouts that are strictly arm specific are a waste of time for most guys.

The reason is your hormonal system. You generate the most testosterone by activating the most muscle mass, and testosterone is the hormone most closely associated with muscle growth. This is why some trainers say that if you want big arms, you should do squats. Squats won't build big arms directly, since they're lower-body exercises. They do use more muscle mass than any other traditional gym exercise, so they generate more testosterone.

Your arm muscles, on the other hand, are relatively small. Even though it feels like you're working hard as hell when you do intense sets of biceps curls and triceps extensions—even though your heart races, your breathing gets ragged, and your forehead pours sweat—you're not really giving your body the stimulus it needs to release its primary muscle-building hormones.

The guys who benefit from arm-exclusive workouts are either bodybuilders who get all the testosterone they need from external sources (sorry, there's that s word again) or guys who have the overall size and strength they want and just want to make subtle changes in arm size.

Myth: I do pushups and pullups, so I don't need to do arm-specific exercises.

Fact: If you want your arms to develop to their full potential, you do have to include isolation exercises in your workouts.

Though pushups and pullups are great exercises, in these movements, your arms are secondary—not primary—muscles. Their job is to help your chest in pushups and your back in pullups. Though your arms still get a great workout, nothing beats triceps extensions and biceps curls for their ability to isolate arm muscles and work them with almost no help from other body parts.

A secondary issue is the number of repetitions you can do per set. Most guys can do quite a few pushups—30 or more per set. However, the ideal muscle-building range is 8 to 12 repetitions per set. Once you go past 12 reps, your body is increasing endurance without adding size. The opposite problem kicks in with pullups. Few guys can knock out sets of 8 to 12 reps. Though sets of 1 to 6 reps build strength, they aren't ideal for increasing muscle mass.

So continue doing those exercises if you like them (especially pullups, which are considered the best exercise for developing your middle- and upper-back muscles). You also have to do the exercises in the Core Program if you want bigger arm muscles.

Myth: It takes lots of volume—for biceps and triceps exercises, 10 to 15 sets each—to build impressive arms.

Fact: Quality matters more than quantity.

One of the biggest and most contentious debates in exercise-science circles is single-set versus multiple-set training. One camp says you can get virtually all the benefits of an exercise from one set in which you exert an all-out effort. The other side says that one set is fine for beginners but more advanced exercisers need to do more to get bigger and stronger.

Dozens of studies have shown the two systems dead even in building both size and strength, while only a handful have shown the multiple-set system to be superior. So is this entire debate the exercise equivalent of the 2000 presidential election, in which there's no clear winner so you just pick the side you want to win and therefore insist that it's made the best case?

No. Most guys will get the best results using a multiple-set system simply because few guys can walk into the gym and do one set of each exercise with enough intensity to make continual gains. Most of us need one to two sets just to prepare our muscles and nerves for an all-out effort. That's why the Core Program will always start you off with one set of each exercise, then move you up to multiple sets.

Getting back to the original question, do you need to do humongous volume—10 or 15 or even 20 sets per muscle group—to make gains? No. Remember, biceps and triceps are small muscle groups. You should be able to give them a complete workout with six sets each, maximum.

Myth: Since arms are small muscles, they should always be trained last in the workout.

Fact: Your workout should start with the muscles you're most interested in building.

It's true that most of your workouts over the course of a year should use the principle of biggest to smallest. Generally, do the exercises that involve the most muscle mass—squats, bench presses, rows—first in your workouts, and the ones for smaller muscles like arms, abdominals, and calves at the end.

However, when you want to improve a particular muscle more than the others, you should train that one first, when your muscles are freshest. If you always work your arms or abdominals when you're already tired from doing squats and bench presses, you'll never train them with all-out effort. The 6-week Core Program will allow you to give your arms the attention they deserve.

Just remember that no exercise system works forever. No matter how great a program you're on, your body eventually gets used to it and figures out how to do it with progressively less effort, involving progressively fewer muscle fibers. Your brain gets bored, too, and you start zoning out in the middle of your workouts, coasting through them and working with progressively less intensity. As a result, you'll start to see diminishing returns. The next step is no returns, and the final step is a return to your original untrained state.

Myth: If I train my biceps and triceps, I don't need to work my forearms.

Fact: Your forearms, like every other muscle, need to be trained with movements that make them the primary mover.

You're only as strong as your weakest link. If your forearms aren't as strong as they should be relative to your bigger muscles, they limit the amount of weight you can lift, no matter what exercise you're doing. To pick just one example, many guys can't work their back muscles with full intensity because their forearms give out too soon on rows and lat pulldowns, forcing them to end their sets before their back muscles reach the point of exhaustion. So the strength you gain from forearm-specific exercises, such as those in the Core Program, will ultimately help you build a stronger chest and back. Try to include forearm exercises in your training a few weeks each year to make sure those smaller muscles keep pace with the rest of your body.

Myth: Pumped-up arms are just for vanity. I don't need them to play sports.

Fact: Any athlete who plays a sport that requires him to use his arms should do specific exercises targeting them (and even soccer players have to be able to rip off their jerseys after a goal).

In some sports, overall size and power do matter more than anything else. Those who play them should spend the majority of their training time doing exercises that develop those traits. Having said that, arm exercises are still important. Stronger biceps help you pull down an opponent (if you're a wrestler or linebacker, for example), while stronger triceps help you throw a ball or swing a bat or racquet. And stronger forearms help anyone who has to grip anything or grapple with anyone.

It's even more crucial to develop muscle balance to prevent injuries. Arm muscles in general—and biceps tendons in particular—are easily and often injured in many sports. Strengthening them is the first and most important step in limiting injuries.

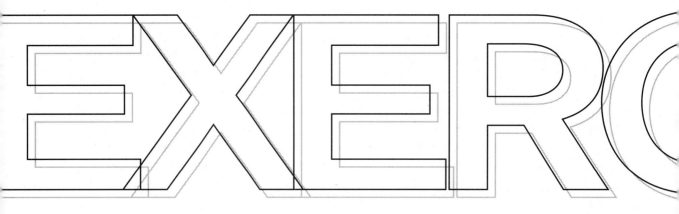

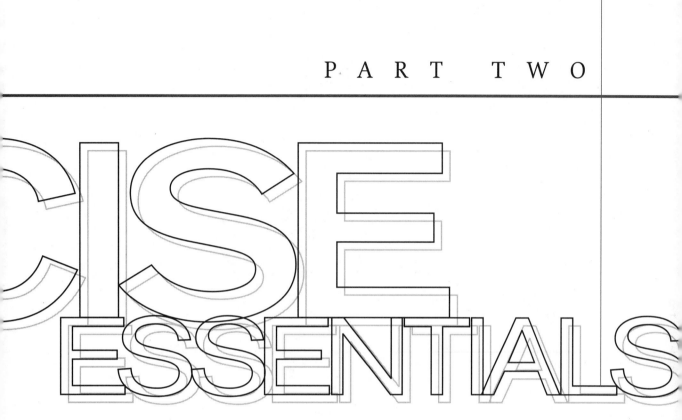

CISE
ESSENTIALS

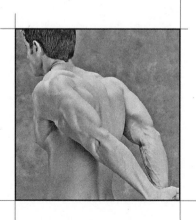

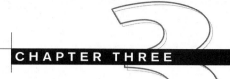

CHAPTER THREE

ESSENTIAL AEROBICS

Since you're reading a book called *Essential Arms*, chances are good that you'd rather toss around some iron than put in heart-quickening miles on a treadmill or stationary bike. Weight training does confer benefits on your heart, the biggest being that it prepares your ticker for extreme exertion. Series of strenuous lifts lasting a half-minute to a minute are good practice for tasks like snow shoveling, wood chopping, carrying boxes up stairs, pushing cars out of snow banks. How important is that? Consider that more people die while shoveling snow than while doing any other form of exercise or household chore.

One 1987 study showed that bodybuilders have lower blood pressures and maximum heart rates during exertion than untrained subjects have. Other studies have also shown an increase in stroke volume, the amount of blood that your heart pumps with each beat. The more blood your heart can pump, the fewer beats it needs to keep your body running, and the less worn out it gets.

Another huge heart benefit of pumping iron is your change in body composition, or your body's ratio of fat to muscle and other tissue. A good weight-lifting program increases your muscle mass, leading to increased metabolism (the speed at which you burn calories while at rest). That helps wipe out body fat, and a leaner, more muscular body makes it easier for your heart to do its job.

LIFE SUPPORT

Now let's look at what weight lifting won't do for your heart.

The most commonly used indicator of cardiovascular fitness is maximum oxygen consumption, or max VO_2. Studies show that weight lifters have average to above-average max VO_2. In other words, their hours in the gym don't give them any great cardio advantage over untrained people. (Nor do those hours give them any disadvantage.)

That being the case, it's best to supplement your weight training with some cardio work. The American College of Sports Medicine recommends a minimum of 30 minutes of cardio exercise, three times a week. At least 20 minutes of that should be spent in your target heart-rate zone.

Your target heart-rate zone is 65 to 85 percent of your maximum heart rate. Your maximum is roughly estimated by subtracting your age from 220. So if you're 30 years old, your estimated maximum heart rate is 190. Your target heart-rate zone is 65 to 85 percent of that, or between 123 and 161 beats per minute.

If you belong to a gym or own a high-end cardio machine with a heart-rate monitor, keeping track of your beats per minute is easy. You just grip whatever the cardio machine tells you to grip, and in a few seconds the machine tells you how fast your heart is beating.

Otherwise, you have to take your pulse at your wrist or neck. The easiest way to do this is to count your heartbeats for 10 seconds and multiply by six.

THE HEART OF THE MATTER

A good cardio workout should include a 5-minute warmup, 20 minutes in your target heart-rate zone, and a 5-minute cooldown. The warmup is just your chosen aerobic activity done at a moderate pace. If you're jogging, for example, you could do a brisk walk as a warmup. The object is to gradually increase your intensity until you hit your target heart-rate zone. Your body needs that time to increase its core temperature, add lubrication to your joints, and prepare your body's chemistry for a shift to exercise.

The cooldown is the same process in reverse. You gradually allow your heart rate to slow until it's closer to its normal speed. Stopping suddenly can leave blood pooled in your extremities, a recipe for a heart attack.

BENEFITS OF AEROBIC EXERCISE

- ■ A stronger heart
- ■ Lower body weight
- ■ Lower resting heart rate, meaning that for most of the day your heart does less work than it would if it weren't fit
- ■ Improved circulation throughout your body
- ■ Decreased blood pressure
- ■ Longer life

ESSENTIAL
PHYSIOLOGY

The basic functions of your arm muscles are pretty simple. Your biceps bend your elbow. Your triceps straighten your elbow. Class dismissed.

Indeed, that's enough knowledge to get you started on the path toward beefing up your arms. But there are subtleties. Your arm muscles also play some supporting roles that may surprise you, and knowing what those are will help you build up the muscles more effectively.

YOUR MUSCLES

Biceps brachii. This is the world's most flexed muscle, and one of the body's simplest. As the prefix *bi* implies, it has two parts, or heads. The long head, on the outside of your arm, crosses the shoulder joint, while the short head, on the inside of your arm, stops just short of your shoulder. Together, the two heads act as one to pull your forearm bones toward your shoulder as well as perform some minor functions that will be discussed later in this chapter.

The long head creates the peak that crowns the best-developed biceps, while the short head lends thickness and determines the length of the muscle. Guys tend to obsess over these aesthetic details (typical letter to a bodybuilding magazine: "How do I make my biceps longer? Help!"). This preoccupation is futile because, for the most part, the

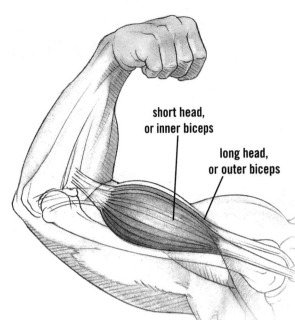

short head, or inner biceps

long head, or outer biceps

The brachialis has the same primary function as the biceps—bending the elbow—without any secondary functions. If your body were a construction crew, the brachialis would be the guy whose only job is to carry the really heavy stuff.

The brachioradialis, on the other hand, is one of the arm's most visible muscles. It's the biggest forearm muscle, and you can see it on skinny fourth-graders (even on skinny fourth-grade girls). It's not a big vanity muscle—the phrase "I'm working my brachioradialis today" has never been overheard in an American gym, to our knowledge—but it still grows along with your brachialis, whether you think about it or not.

length of your biceps is genetically determined. Some exercise scientists—and most muscleheads—believe that a process called hyperplasia occurs, in which muscle cells split and form new cells in response to intense, targeted exercise. Thus, if you want your biceps to be longer, you continually target your inner biceps, set after set, workout after workout, until your body spackles new muscle cells on top of the old ones to push the lower edge of the muscle closer to the elbow joint. The majority of scientists, however, view the idea of hyperplasia with skepticism.

Brachialis and brachioradialis. The brachialis is a thick, strong muscle that you won't see on your own arm until you're in top shape. It rests between the upper-arm bone and the biceps brachii, and for it to be visible, you have to be very lean and extremely muscular. When you do build it up, the result will be obvious: It will push the biceps upward, creating a higher peak on your outer arm.

Triceps brachii. These muscles actually comprise about two-thirds of your upper-arm mass, even though a much smaller fraction of your vanity is tied up in them. *Tri* refers to the fact that the muscle has

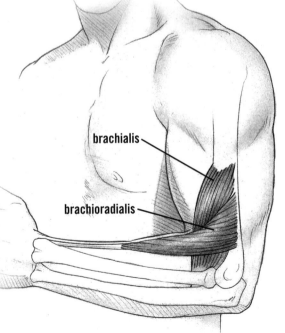

brachialis

brachioradialis

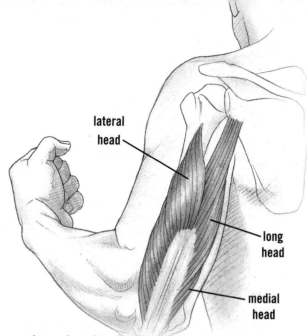

lateral
head

long
head

medial
head

ample—and play important roles in sports. Hitting a backhand in tennis or racquetball may be the best example.

BODY MECHANICS

Your arm muscles are unique in that, from day one of an exercise program, you can feel exactly when you're working them. By contrast, it may take weeks or months before you become familiar with the feeling of exerting your chest, back, or shoulder muscles. But the sensations in your arm muscles can be illusory—even when you feel a burn in your triceps or a pump in your biceps, you have no idea if you're successfully isolating the muscles. And make no mistake, the key to successfully building the muscles is isolating them in arm-specific exercises. This section will give you a better idea of how to pull off that trick and get the best results.

three heads: the long head, which is on the inside of your arm; the lateral head, which is on the outside; and the medial head, which lies underneath the long head. The long and lateral heads combine to form the horseshoe shape you see on the best-developed triceps.

Forearm flexors. The muscles on the inside of your forearm include the flexor carpi radialis, flexor carpi ulnaris, and palmaris longus. Though these muscles are small, they offer big help in exercises like biceps curls and lat pulldowns, and they are crucial in sports. They play a role in throwing a baseball or football and in swinging a tennis racket or baseball bat. Mark McGwire's forearms are exhibit A.

Forearm extensors. On the outside of your forearm are the extensor carpi radialis longus and extensor carpi radialis brevis. Like the forearm flexors, they act as supporting and stabilizing muscles in a number of popular gym exercises—bench presses and triceps extensions, for ex-

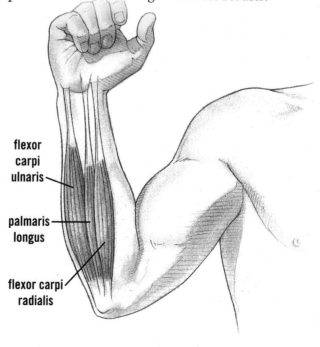

flexor
carpi
ulnaris

palmaris
longus

flexor carpi
radialis

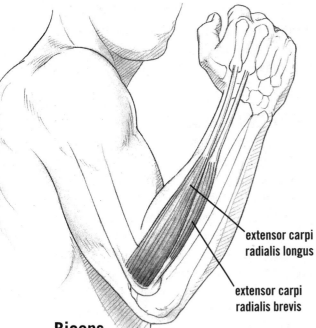

extensor carpi
radialis longus

extensor carpi
radialis brevis

Biceps

What you do: When you emphasize your biceps, you bring your forearm closer to your shoulder. It doesn't matter what position your arm is in when you begin this movement—it could be overhead, as when you're doing a chinup (1), or hanging straight down, as in a biceps curl (2).

You can selectively emphasize the inner or outer head of the biceps by changing a few variables. If you use a wide grip on a barbell biceps curl, you'll work the inner head more intensely. The narrower your grip, the more you'll work the outer head. Also, if you do dumbbell curls while lying on your back on an incline bench, you'll work your outer head preferentially.

Other biceps actions: The biceps are also responsible for a movement called supination, in which you rotate your forearm from a neutral position (palms facing each other) to a palms-up, or supinated, position. Finally, the biceps assist in

raising your arm out in front of your body, although the front part of the shoulder muscle is the primary mover in that action.

Brachialis and Brachioradialis

What you do: These muscles bend your elbow when your palm is either facing down or in a neutral position. The hammer curl is the best example (3).

Other brachialis and brachioradialis actions: There really aren't any for the brachialis, but the brachioradialis is more versatile. It also helps rotate your forearm inward (supination) and outward (pronation).

Triceps

What you do: You increase the distance between your forearm and upper arm—in other words, you straighten your arm when it's bent (4). It doesn't matter whether your arm is down at your side or overhead when you begin this action.

Other triceps actions: The long head of the triceps also helps bring your arm down to your side from an overhead position, though the latissimus dorsi—the large fan-shaped muscles in your middle back—are the primary movers in that action, with help from your chest muscles.

Forearm Flexors

What you do: You bend your wrist so your palm moves toward your inner forearm. The wrist curl is the best example (5).

Other forearm flexor actions: These muscles assist the biceps in bending your

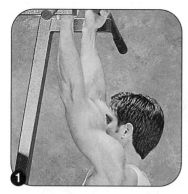

Biceps brachii

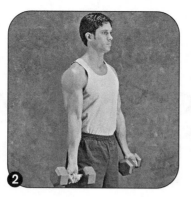

Biceps brachii

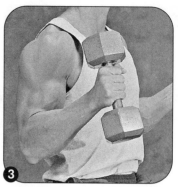

Brachialis and brachioradialis

elbow. In high-repetition sets of back and biceps exercises, you may feel the burn in your forearm flexors before you feel it in the muscles you're actually targeting. They're also the muscles charged with waving bye-bye: When you hold up your forearm and move your hand from side to side, you use your forearm flexors. There's another, more private, activity in which forearm flexors play a prominent role. Let's just say that if you do this too often, you risk overdevelopment of the forearm flexors in your dominant arm. If anyone notices, tell them you've become really fond of tennis.

Forearm Extensors

What you do: You bend your wrist so the back of your hand moves toward your outer forearm, as in a reverse wrist curl (6).

Other forearm extensor actions: These muscles have a minor role in straightening your arm when it's bent. Chances are, though, you'll barely notice that they're in action when you're doing exercises for your triceps.

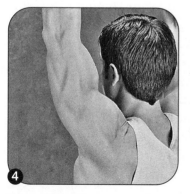

Triceps brachii

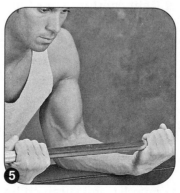

Forearm flexors

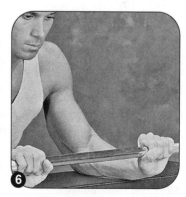

Forearm extensors

5

ESSENTIAL FLEXIBILITY
STRETCHES

STRETCHING
STRATEGIES

Stretch to a point of mild discomfort and no farther.

Hold each stretch for 20 to 30 seconds.

Breathe as you stretch.

Hold steady—don't bounce. If your muscle softens, you can move deeper into the stretch. But don't push into pain. That defeats the purpose.

Don't stretch as a warmup or when your body is cold.

Stretch at least three times a week.

Tune in. Pay attention to how your muscles feel and perform as you stretch. You can daydream at work—good stretches require focus.

Guys rarely stretch. More important, guys rarely enjoy stretching, which explains why so few bother with it.

But how much would you enjoy needing two tries to get out of an armchair? Grunting like a sea elephant when you bend down to pick up the newspaper in your driveway? Uttering the phrase, "Oh, it's my damned back again" when asked why you resemble a human question mark?

A tight body can compromise your health and happiness in any number of ways. Here are just a few.

■ Tight calves and Achilles tendons can lead to knee injuries.

■ Tight hamstrings or hip flexors (the muscles on the front of your pelvis) can pull your lower back out of its natural alignment, causing chronic problems.

■ Tight chest muscles can round your shoulders forward, leading to chronic upper-back discomfort.

■ Tight arm muscles can decrease your range of motion on biceps and triceps exercises, eventually leading to shortened muscles.

■ Tight muscles and connective tissues anywhere on your body can hamper your ability to play any sport, from golf to basketball to skiing. And an inflexible body is more easily injured in sports, leading to considerable time on the DL due to torn muscles and sprained ligaments.

The antidote is simple: Stretch. The following stretches should take you about 5 minutes. It's best to do them when your body is already warmed up. So do them after your warmup and before your weight-lifting workout. It's also okay to do them after your workout, although that makes it much easier to skip them altogether. You give a greater effort to pre-workout stretching because your body is warmed up and ready to work, rather than tired and ready to hit the showers.

Triceps

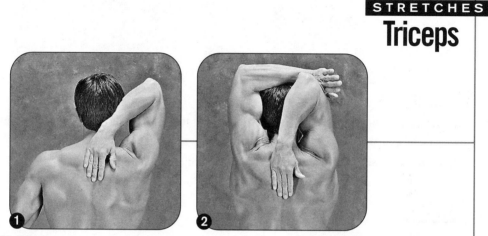

READY, SET, GO:

1. Lift your right arm so your elbow is next to your right ear, with your elbow bent and your right hand on the middle of your back.

2. Cross your left arm over your head so the back of your left hand lies against your right triceps muscle. Push back with your left hand until you feel a stretch in your right triceps. Repeat to your left side.

Biceps and Forearm Flexors

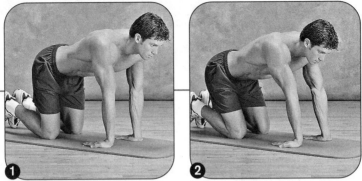

READY, SET, GO:

1. Kneel on the floor with your palms on the floor in front of you, directly in line with your shoulders, and your fingers pointing back toward you.

2. Lean back until you feel a gentle stretch in your biceps and forearms.

Neck

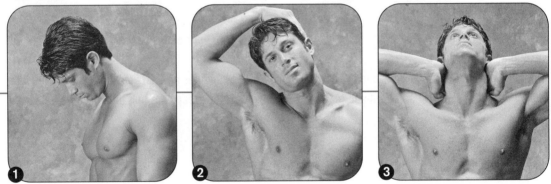

READY, SET, GO:

1. Drop your head forward, chin to chest.

2. Place your right hand on the left side of your head, just above your ear. Lower your right ear toward your right shoulder, using your hand to gently assist. Repeat to your left side.

3. Place your hands behind your neck with your fingertips touching, and gently tilt your head back, using your hands for support. Don't crunch your neck back and compress your vertebrae.

Shoulders

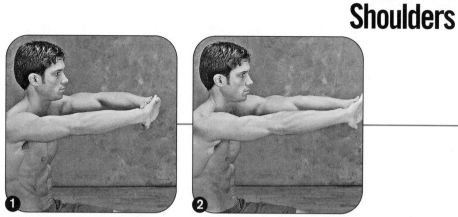

Chest

READY, SET, GO:

1. Extend your arms in front of your body, interlocking your fingers and turning your palms away from you.

2. Round your upper back as you press your palms outward.

READY, SET, GO:

1. Clasp your hands behind your lower back.

2. Slowly extend your hands up and back.

Abdomen

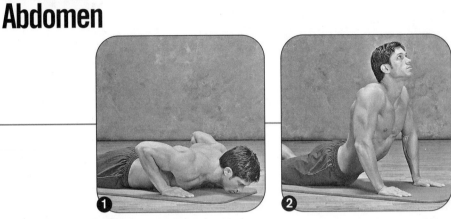

READY, SET, GO:

1. Lie on your stomach with your hands directly below your shoulders, palms down.

2. Slowly push up with your arms, arching your torso up. Keep your hips on the floor, and look up.

Lower Back and Gluteals

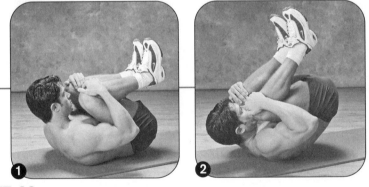

READY, SET, GO:

1. Lie flat on your back and bring both knees to your chest. Grab both knees and gently pull them toward your shoulders. At the same time, tuck your head and bring your chin to your chest.

2. Gently and slowly, roll back and forth five times. *Caution:* You need a mat or well-padded and carpeted floor to do this safely.

Groin

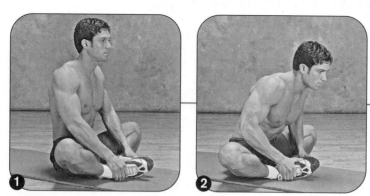

READY, SET, GO:

1. Sit on the floor and place the soles of your feet together in front of you.

2. Lean forward until you feel a gentle stretch in your groin.

Quadriceps (Front Thighs) and Hip Flexors

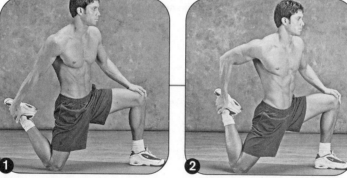

READY, SET, GO:

1. Kneel on your right knee, with your left foot flat on the floor in front of you. Reach back and grab the top of your right foot.

2. Lean forward until you feel a gentle stretch in the front of your right thigh and the right side of your pelvis. Repeat to your left side.

Lower-Back and Hamstrings

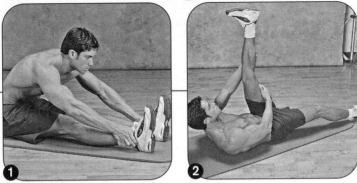

READY, SET, GO:

1. Sit on the floor and extend both legs out in front of you. Lean forward and lightly grasp your knees with your elbows pointed out. As you become more flexible, try to grasp farther down your legs (grasp your calves, ankles, or feet).

2. Lie on your back, lift your left leg, and grab it with both hands, either just below your knee or just above it—whichever is more comfortable. Gently pull it toward your head. You may find it helpful to raise your head, bringing your chin to your chest. Repeat with your right leg.

Lower Back

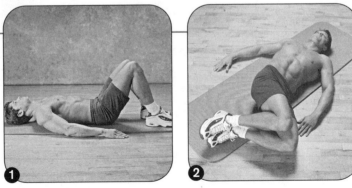

READY, SET, GO:

1. Lie on your back with your knees bent and your feet flat on the floor.

2. Let both legs fall to your left side. Repeat to your right side.

CHAPTER SIX

ESSENTIAL
PRINCIPLES

This book gives you a lot of technical information about the anatomy of your arms, the proper way to lift a weight, and how many times you should do each exercise. None of this information will help you build muscle, though, if your overall approach to training is wrong.

Here are four basic training principles to help you get the results you want from your arms buildup.

PRINCIPLE #1:
CONSISTENTLY CHANGE

Most guys make little if any progress beyond what they achieve in their first year or two of lifting. Part of the problem is just the way muscles work: They don't keep growing forever. Eventually, your body hits its genetic limit, and only drastic measures (usually of the pharmacological variety) will move it past that point.

But very few guys ever truly hit that limit. Most simply stop giving their muscles any new stimuli. Your body needs you to force it to adapt to something different—new exercises and routines, heavier weights, different lifting speeds.

The Core Program addresses this issue by introducing new challenges every week for 6 weeks. Once you complete the program, you'll need to maintain that same pace of change.

(continued on page 38)

Variety is the key to increasing strength and muscle size, but only if it's the right kind of variety. Here are some of the variables you can manipulate to help you make consistent improvements.

Volume. The simplest way to measure this is by the number of sets you perform in a workout. A low-volume routine might involve 1 set of each of eight exercises. A high-volume routine might be more than 24 sets in a workout—more than 3 sets of eight different exercises. In the 6-week Core Program, you start off with a very low-volume routine and move up to higher volume—in the final workout, you do 11 exercises and a total of 20 sets.

Each extreme has its merits. Low-volume routines are great for beginners, for guys coming back from injuries or long layoffs, for guys who are so busy that they're more worried about maintenance than about improvement. But no one can stay on a low-volume routine for long and expect to see big gains.

Conversely, a high-volume routine is usually the best way for advanced lifters to make gains. If 12 or 15 or 20 sets per workout don't produce gains, they try 24 or 30 sets.

But more work doesn't always translate into more results. Often, it has the opposite effect: You get injured or burned out. Varying your workout volume throughout the year helps keep you motivated. When you're in a low-volume stage, you leave the gym each day looking forward to your next workout since you haven't fully taxed your body. And when you hit the highest-volume stage, you know you have to beat yourself up like this for only a few weeks before easing up again.

Intensity. There are a few ways to define intensity, but in this case, it refers to the amount of weight lifted. The closer you are to the absolute maximum weight you can lift once, the higher your intensity.

Maximum muscle growth is thought to occur when you work with weights that are between 60 and 80 percent of your one-repetition maximum. So if the most weight you can bench-press once is 200 pounds, you'll build muscle best when you work with between 120 and 160 pounds.

At this intensity, most guys can do sets of 8 to 20 repetitions. Generally, if you can only do sets of fewer than 8 repetitions, you're working with more than 80 percent of your one-rep maximum. That will lead to the biggest strength gains but not necessarily to the biggest improvement in muscle size.

Your body makes the best improvements when you vary intensity throughout the year, sometimes doing high-repetition sets with lighter weights, sometimes doing low-repetition sets with maximal weights.

Order of exercises. There is no one perfect way to arrange the exercises in your workout. In the Core Program, you'll do arm exercises first in your workout, before exercising any other body parts. Most exercise books and magazines have you work the biggest muscles in your body first. The only hard-and-fast rule is that you should vary the order throughout the year, sometimes starting with arms, as in this program; sometimes starting with your chest, as when you're trying to improve your maximum bench press; sometimes starting with legs, as when you're trying to improve your vertical jump for basketball.

But even if your goal throughout the year is simply to get into better shape, you still need to change the order of exercises occasionally. If you always do certain exercises last, you'll always do them when you're already tired from other exercises, so you'll never get the full benefit from them.

Repetition speed. This is a relatively new addition to the list of strength-training variables. Most guys lift at just one speed, taking 1 second to lift the weight and 2 seconds to lower it. But fitness trainers have discovered that by deliberately speeding up or slowing down repetition speeds, you can get different results from the same exercises.

The Core Program recommends that you lift the weight for 1 second, pause, lower it for 2 or 3 seconds, pause, and then lift again. But in other programs, you should try different speeds. If you're an athlete, you may want to lift the weights faster to improve your muscles' power. If your main focus is building bigger muscles, you want to lift slower—taking a full 4 or 5 seconds to lower the weight, for example—to keep your muscles under tension longer. Several studies have shown that the lowering portion of the lift is tougher on your muscles than the lifting phase. Extending that lowering phase thus produces greater gains in muscle size.

Rest periods. **The amount of rest you take between sets has an effect on how your body reacts to each exercise.**

■ No rest. Some people do circuit workouts, in which they go from one exercise to another with little or no rest between sets. This isn't a good strategy for building muscle size, but it increases muscular endurance and overall stamina. And it certainly burns calories.

■ Short rest: 30 to 60 seconds. When you do higher-repetition sets, your muscles recover quickly between sets. Resting for 60 seconds may be the best strategy for improving your body's ratio of muscle to fat. Studies show that your body burns mostly fat calories between sets, so if you lift for 30 to 60 seconds and then rest for 30 to 60 seconds, you'll burn more fat calories than if you went from one exercise to another with no rest.

■ Moderate rest: 90 to 120 seconds. When you start using heavier weights and doing sets of fewer than 10 repetitions, you need this much time to allow your muscles and nerves to regroup between sets. This is hardly wasted time. When your muscles fully recover between sets, you're able to perform more repetitions with heavier weights—and thus build bigger muscles.

■ Long rest: 2 to 5 minutes. Sets using maximal weights require maximal recovery in between. The benefit to waiting this long is the tremendous strength gains you'll make. For example, if you do sets of one to five repetitions, your only goal is to use the heaviest possible weight in each set. Getting incomplete rest between sets means you have to use less weight or do fewer repetitions.

TAKE THE BEST, IGNORE THE REST

How do you know if a routine is appropriate for you or if the advice you're getting is good or garbage? It's hard, but here are a few guidelines.

■ If you're a beginner, your routine should be low volume: one or two sets of 8 to 12 exercises, two or three times a week, tops. Research has shown that beginners get the same gains from low-volume routines as from high-volume ones. Minimum volume also allows you to build strength and resilience in your joints and connective tissues with little risk of injury. So if someone suggests that you launch into an elaborate program of hour-long workouts four or five times a week, they don't know what they're talking about.

■ If you're trying to lose weight, you need a routine that focuses on your biggest muscles, particularly those in your lower body. Working and building those muscles speeds up your metabolism and produces faster weight loss. Routines that focus on smaller muscles are a big waste of time for you.

BE EFFECTIVE AND EFFICIENT

The goal of an exercise program isn't to spend so much time at the gym that you need to have your mail forwarded there. Having strong, muscled arms is pretty pointless if there's no time left over to use

them—to help the neighbor push his stalled car, to toss a giggling kid into the air, to carry a comely woman off to the bedroom. Plus, you probably have less time for exercise—and for everything else—than ever before: By one estimate, Americans each work 8 more weeks a year than we did 20 years ago.

Limiting the length of your workouts not only will give you some of your life back but also will maximize your fitness benefits. That's because the longer you exercise, the more catabolic, or muscle-wasting, hormones your body produces. These counteract the anabolic, or muscle-building, hormones you produce while lifting weights.

Most experts recommend that you keep your weight workouts under 1 hour. If you can't perform your workout in less than an hour, there's probably something wrong with it. You're doing too many sets of too many exercises (or spending too much time checking out the Pilates bodies). You won't have this problem with the workouts in the Core Program; but when you complete the program and move on to other routines, you may find yourself suffering "workout bloat": You'll know so many great exercises that you'll try to do them all in every workout. Here are a couple of ways to avoid getting bloated.

Divide your program into two, three, or four separate workouts. The easiest way to do this is to split up your upper-body and lower-body exercises and perform each workout once or twice a week. But you could also use three separate workouts (one for back and biceps, one for lower body, and one for chest, shoulders, and triceps, for example) or even four (one for chest and back, one for lower-body exercises that primarily use the quadriceps, one for shoulders and arms, and one for lower-body exercises that focus on the hamstrings) and do each once a week.

Eliminate redundant exercises. Some guys do three or four sets of three or four different exercises for each muscle group—most of which are probably wasted effort. If you do the first exercise with enough intensity, you probably won't get much additional benefit from subsequent exercises.

PRINCIPLE #4:
TAKE BREAKS

Once you start seeing results from your workout program, the last thing you want to do is take a week off. But you have to give your body an occasional break. Some trainers even recommend taking off one week every month. That's right—three weeks of workouts followed by a week without workouts.

What these trainers have discovered is that your body makes its best gains when it's given enough time to recover. Conversely, training hard for months on end without recovery time produces one of three results: (1) no gains, since your body is too exhausted to improve, (2) injury, since most workouts are based on repetitive movements that wear down muscles and joints if you never take a break, and (3) burnout, since anything taken to an extreme produces mental as well as physical fatigue.

The best way to integrate rest into the 6-week Core Program is to take off for a full week after completing it. Here are a few other rules of recovery that are built into the Core Program. You should apply them to any workout regimen.

■ Take at least a full-day break every week.
■ Limit your weight workouts to four a week, tops. (The Core Program calls for two or three, but many guys do as many as six.)
■ Take a full week off from weight lifting every 4 to 8 weeks or anytime you complete a major program.

7

ESSENTIAL
TECHNIQUES

xercise is a lot like sex: You can do it for a lifetime and still find new ways to get better results. Even better, you don't have to be an expert on the subject to get started—though it does help to know the basics before you jump in. A little knowledge up front can save you a lot of grief down the road. With sex, you know what kind of grief can result. ("Hi, Daddy!" is only one example from a list.) The information in this chapter will help you avoid the two major exercise pitfalls: disappointing results and injury. It will help you to continually make improvements and spare yourself the downtime that accompanies a pulled muscle or strained ligament. Here are seven rules of arm exercise.

#1
WARM UP FIRST

You walk into the gym, pick up a barbell, and start pumping out some biceps curls. You set down the barbell, grab some dumbbells, and start knocking out some triceps extensions. No, you didn't warm up. But what's the problem? It's not as if your arms fell off or anything.

Here's the problem—actually, two problems. First, cold muscles can't work as efficiently as warm muscles. So you won't be able to use as much weight or do as many repetitions with a given weight as you could have if you'd warmed up. Second, unprepared muscles and connective tissues are more easily strained or torn.

A warmup is a two-part process. The first step is simply and literally raising your core body temperature. You can accomplish this with any type of moderately intense activity; it doesn't even have to be formal exercise. It could be a few minutes of yard work or playing with your kids. (But don't think that you can warm up just by taking a hot shower. That only raises your skin temperature; your core temperature remains unchanged.) Start your warmup slowly, and gradually increase your pace. You should feel it in your skin, as you break a light sweat.

The second part of a warmup is moving the specific muscles and joints you're going to work. This shunts blood from your gut, where it's being used to keep your internal organs functioning, to your arms. It also prompts your joints to release a protective coating called synovial fluid. This is just like warming up your car on a cold morning. You want the oil to work its way into the pistons before you drive off. Your wrists, elbows, and shoulders deserve the same courtesy.

For the Core Program, a set of biceps exercises plus a set of triceps exercises, each using about half to two-thirds of your starting weight, will do the trick. So if you're going to do your first exercise with 20-pound dumbbells, use 10 to 15 pounds for your warmup. Do the warmup sets slowly, completing the same number of repetitions that you'll do in your workout sets. Then, rest your muscles for a minute between your warmup sets and your first workout set.

#2
GO THROUGH ALL THE MOTIONS
Muscles adapt to the tasks that you impose upon them. If you always work them

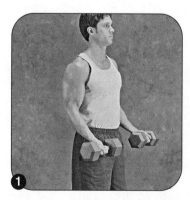 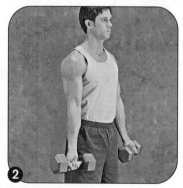

To get the greatest benefits from your workout, you have to do each repetition through your complete range of motion. For instance, lowering your arms only 135 degrees during a biceps curl (1) works fewer muscle fibers than extending them a full 180 degrees (2).

through an abbreviated range of motion, they adapt by getting stronger only within that range of motion, plus about 15 degrees. It's tempting to progressively shorten your range as you get more experienced in the weight room—you can lift a lot more weight if you don't have to lift it as far. But you ultimately cut short your gains because you leave lots of muscle fibers unworked. If you don't work them, they don't grow. Eventually, they'll disappear, and your muscles will be permanently shorter.

It's simple to work your arm muscles through the full range. Lower the weights as far as you can on each repetition, pause, then start the next repetition. Increase the amount of weight only when you can do all the recommended repetitions in your sets through this full range of motion.

#3
TAKE THE NEGATIVE ALONG WITH THE POSITIVE

If you've never lifted weights before, you'll quickly discover that certain parts of an exercise are much easier than others. The reason is that gravity has different effects at different points in your range of motion. For example, the first few inches of a biceps curl are easy because you're moving the weights out, not up. You could do those first few inches forever and not gain anything, other than perhaps some grip strength from holding the weights. As soon as you start to lift up the weights, you're working against gravity. That's when you start building muscle.

You also work against gravity when you lower the weights. This is called the negative portion of the exercise, and it's even more taxing for your muscles than the lifting, or positive, phase. Most guys skip this phase altogether and just let gravity take over. But you'll build more muscle, and build it faster, if you consciously control the weights throughout the exercise. A good technique to master is counting to three during the negative phase of each repetition.

#4
KEEP BREATHING

Most guys, when they first start lifting weights, have to be reminded to breathe on each repetition. You want to exhale as you complete the repetition, and then inhale as you lower the weight. But it's not a problem if you do it backward. The point is to avoid holding your breath through a series of repetitions. That can cause your blood pressure to spike upward.

#5
ALWAYS CHOOSE QUALITY OVER QUANTITY

The weight you use on curls and extensions is simply a tool. A carpenter doesn't assume that using a bigger hammer will ensure that he builds a better house. It's the same with a barbell or dumbbells: Bigger weights don't automatically translate to better muscles. First, you need to master tips 1 through 4—warming up, completing your range of motion, working against gravity, and breathing. Only then should you worry about increasing weight.

Quality is an elusive target because you have to work to achieve it on each repetition. Each rep should look perfect from the outside and feel perfect from the inside. Anyone watching your workout should see you completing your repetitions smoothly, with each rep as long as the previous one. Interior perfection means that you feel your targeted muscle being flexed throughout the exercise. You know what a flexed muscle feels like—you've been practicing since you were 5.

In the first few repetitions of a set, even though your muscle is flexed, the weight feels light, and you have to overcome the temptation to fling it up and down. In the middle repetitions, the weight feels just right, and you feel as if your muscles were growing right before your eyes. It's in the last repetitions that you have to fight hardest to keep your form. You're tempted to speed up your repetitions and let gravity take over when you lower the weight.

When you can't control these aspects of the repetition anymore, the set is over. You've done your work and fully exhausted your muscles. When they can't do the exercise right anymore, you shouldn't force your muscles to do it wrong.

#6
TAKE THE GOOD WITHOUT THE BAD

At the end of a set, you probably feel pretty damn uncomfortable. Your muscles burn, your arms shake, and your breathing sounds like it did on your wedding night.

That's good pain, and it's pretty much the Holy Grail of muscle building. You don't have to go to this point on every set of every exercise. But when you're focusing on your arm muscles, you'll probably be disappointed if you don't. Walking away from arm exercises without getting that shaking, burning pump is like leaving money on the table in a poker game.

Shooting pains, sharp pains, spasms, and pain that moves beyond the muscles you're exercising are a different story. They're bad pains, and they mean you're hurt. They give you no choice but to stop your set and try to figure out what went wrong.

Manipulate the area where the pain originated—your elbow, shoulder, wrist, or possibly even your back or neck. Move the sore body part through its range of motion, and stretch it. If it starts to swell or is so stiff that you can't work it through its range of motion, you're injured, and your workout is over. If you don't stop and rest, you'll aggravate the injury.

#7
ISOLATE YOUR ARM MUSCLES

The Core Program features mostly isolation exercises for your arms. When you do these exercises, the only joints you should be working are your elbows. If you move any other joints—whether they're your shoulders, wrists, lower back, or hips—you're taking work away from your arm muscles.

Not every exercise is an isolation movement. In Level Three of the Core Program, you'll do bench dips for your triceps that move both your elbows and your shoulders. That's by design. The long head of the triceps muscle crosses the shoulder joint, so multijoint exercises are important when you're trying to fully develop your triceps. Another good multijoint triceps exercise is the close-grip bench press, which will be featured in chapter 13.

When you are doing isolation exercises, make sure you do them right. Here are some good isolation exercises that guys often unintentionally turn into sloppy multijoint exercises.

Overhead Triceps Extension
Problem: You drop your upper arms as you lower the weights, then raise them back in as you raise the weights (3).

The grip you choose affects the way you hit your muscles—a biceps curl becomes a different exercise if you move from a wide grip to a narrow grip or from underhand to overhand. Here are the different ways to grip a barbell or dumbbell and the effect each will have on your quest for bigger arms.

1. This is the standard barbell grip for biceps curls and wrist curls. **It can also be used to change the angle in some triceps, shoulder, and trapezius exercises. When used in triceps exercises, this grip emphasizes the lateral head (the outside of the horseshoe). Usually, your hands should be a little more than shoulder-width apart.**

2. Overhand, or pronated, grip. **This grip is used to emphasize the forearms, brachialis, brachioradialis, and the outer head of the biceps. This is also the standard grip for most barbell triceps exercises as well as chest, shoulder, and trapezius work. Usually, your hands should be slightly farther than shoulder-width apart.**

3. Hammer, or neutral, grip. **When used in biceps ex-**

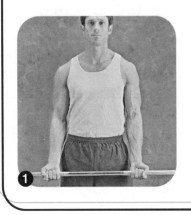

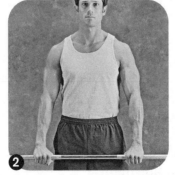

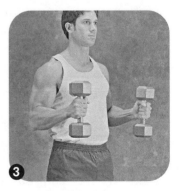

This actually involves two extra joints. First off, dropping your upper arms means you have to use your shoulders to lift them back up again. But you're probably also moving your shoulder blades. This is a separate joint that is responsible

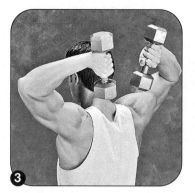
3

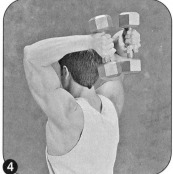
4

ercises, this dumbbell grip emphasizes the outer head of the biceps, along with the brachialis and brachioradialis. For triceps exercises, this grip is usually the standard for ensuring that all three heads of the muscle get a thorough workout, whether it's used with dumbbells, a rope extension on a cable machine, or parallel bars for dips.

4. Wide underhand grip. **You can use this grip for variety, to emphasize the inner head of the biceps. How far apart you place your hands is up to you—anywhere from 4 to 8 inches outside each shoulder is fine.**

5. Narrow underhand grip. **This may be the most beneficial grip for overall biceps development; it hits both**

heads of the biceps and the brachialis. "Narrow" can be defined as anything less than shoulder-width.

6. Narrow overhand, or close, grip. **Usually used for bench presses, this hand position emphasizes the triceps while limiting chest involvement.**

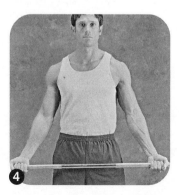
4

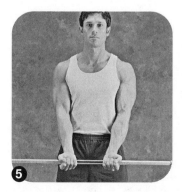
5

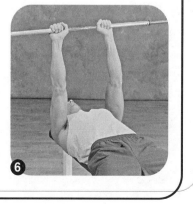
6

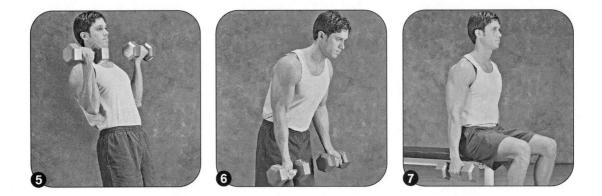

for shrugging your shoulders up and down or squeezing your shoulder blades together in back. The muscle used here is your trapezius, the diamond-shaped muscle in your middle and upper back. The trapezius (or *traps*, in gym-speak) is a perfectly fine muscle, and you definitely want to spend some time building it as you get more experienced in the weight room. But if you're trying to develop your triceps, you don't want your traps to carry the load.

Solution: Imagine that you have a string around your upper arms, making it impossible to move them apart. You want them to stay pointed toward the ceiling throughout the exercise (see photo 4 on the previous page). This takes some getting used to, but if you start with very light weights and work at performing slow, smooth repetitions, you'll be very happy with the results.

Biceps Curls

Problem: You rock back (5) and forth (6) when doing biceps exercises.

Solution: Sit down during dumbbell exercises (7). This makes it much less tempting to bend forward or lean back and makes it impossible to use your knees to generate momentum.

Problem: You move your upper arms

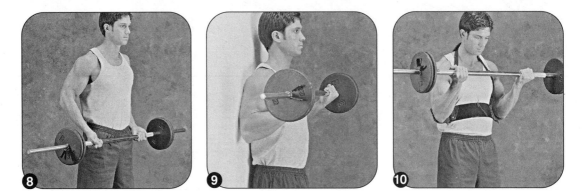

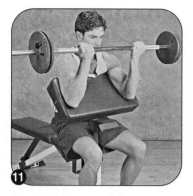

backward so you can lift more weight (8). This problem is difficult to self-diagnose. Chances are, you'll think you're doing everything right until a trainer or friend or even some meddlesome jerk points out that your upper arms look like they're shifting gears on a racecar.

Solution: Rest the backs of your upper arms against a wall (9), arm blaster (10), or a preacher bench (11). The first effect you'll notice is that you can't lift nearly as much weight. The second effect will come a day or two later, when you'll realize that your biceps are more sore than they've ever been. That's the result of truly isolating them.

Don't use a prop all the time; just try it for a few workouts a couple of times a year. The rest of the time, you want to develop this control on your own. But there's nothing like a wall, arm blaster, or preacher bench to remind you how much extra movement you're putting into your biceps exercises, even when you think you're using perfect form.

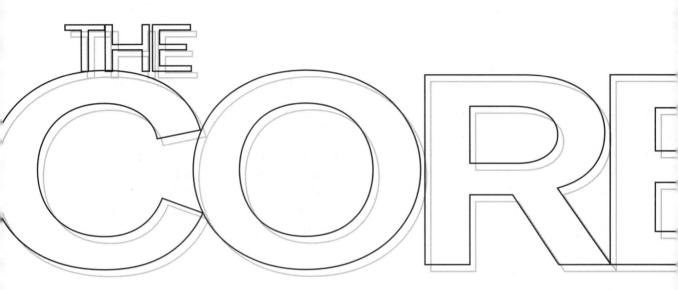

PROGRAM

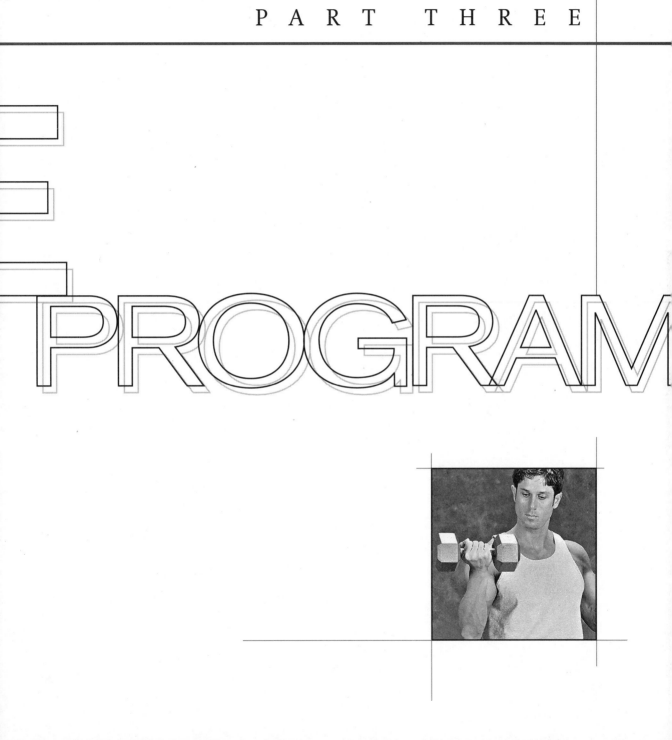

8

ESSENTIAL KNOWLEDGE

The goal of *Essential Arms* is to put you on a structured program designed to build bigger arm muscles. During the 6-week Core Program, you'll lift weights twice a week, adding sets and exercises as you go.

In the first 2 weeks, you'll do arm exercises plus a lower-body strength-training routine. In the next 2 weeks, you'll add more arm exercises, plus an upper-body routine. In the final 2 weeks, you'll do all that plus even more arm exercises. All told, you'll spend about an hour lifting weights, twice a week. Combine that with three half-hour sessions of cardiovascular exercise, and by the end of the Core Program, you can expect to spend 3½ hours a week working out.

As explained in chapter 1, this isn't a book for the Future Nightclub Bouncers of America. The Core Program is a simple and effective way to begin an exercise program or to restart one if you're disappointed with whatever routine you're been doing up till now. But despite its simplicity, there are some sophisticated techniques involved.

You'll start Level One of the Core Program with just four arm exercises, one for biceps, one for triceps, and two for forearms. You'll continue doing those four exercises in the second and third levels. Since you're a beginner, four arm exercises are all you need to help you make anatomical adaptations to strength training. Your body wouldn't de-

(continued on page 54)

Use these charts to help you monitor your progress through the Core Program. In the "Workout" columns, the numbers on the left sides of the slashes are the recom-

WEEK 1		
LEVEL-ONE EXERCISES	**WORKOUT 1**	**WORKOUT 2**
Overhead triceps extension	1 set, 8–12 reps/	1 set, 8–12 reps/
Biceps curl	1 set, 8–12 reps/	1 set, 8–12 reps/
Wrist curl	1 set, 8–12 reps/	1 set, 8–12 reps/
Reverse wrist curl	1 set, 8–12 reps/	1 set, 8–12 reps/
Squat	1 set, 10–15 reps/	1 set, 10–15 reps/
Lunge	1 set, 10–15 reps/	1 set, 10–15 reps/
Calf raise	1 set, 10–15 reps/	1 set, 10–15 reps/
Crunch with a cross	1 set, 10–15 reps/	1 set, 10–15 reps/
Opposite arm and leg raise	1 set, 10–15 reps/	1 set, 10–15 reps/
LEVEL-TWO EXERCISES	**WORKOUT 1**	**WORKOUT 2**
Kickback	1 set, 8–12 reps/	1 set, 8–12 reps/
Overhead triceps extension	1 set, 8–12 reps/	1 set, 8–12 reps/
Hammer curl	1 set, 8–12 reps/	1 set, 8–12 reps/
Biceps curl	1 set, 8–12 reps/	1 set, 8–12 reps/
Wrist curl	1 set, 8–12 reps/	1 set, 8–12 reps/
Reverse wrist curl	1 set, 8–12 reps/	1 set, 8–12 reps/
Bench press	1 set, 8–12 reps/	1 set, 8–12 reps/
Bent-over row	1 set, 8–12 reps/	1 set, 8–12 reps/
Rotation press	1 set, 8–12 reps/	1 set, 8–12 reps/
Squat	1 set, 10–15 reps/	1 set, 10–15 reps/
Lunge	1 set, 10–15 reps/	1 set, 10–15 reps/
Calf raise	1 set, 10–15 reps/	1 set, 10–15 reps/
Crossover	1 set, 10–15 reps/	1 set, 10–15 reps/
Superman	1 set, 10–15 reps/	1 set, 10–15 reps/

mended number of sets and repetitions. Track how many

sets and reps you actually finish by recording those

numbers to the right sides of the slashes.

WEEK 2

WORKOUT 1	WORKOUT 2
2 sets, 8–12 reps/	2 sets, 8–12 reps/
2 sets, 8–12 reps/	2 sets, 8–12 reps/
1 set, 8–12 reps/	1 set, 8–12 reps/
1 set, 8–12 reps/	1 set, 8–12 reps/
2 sets, 10–15 reps/	2 sets, 10–15 reps/
2 sets, 10–15 reps/	2 sets, 10–15 reps/
2 sets, 10–15 reps/	2 sets, 10–15 reps/
2 sets, 10–15 reps/	2 sets, 10–15 reps/
2 sets, 10–15 reps/	2 sets, 10–15 reps/

WORKOUT 1	WORKOUT 2
2 sets, 8–12 reps/	2 sets, 8–12 reps/
2 sets, 8–12 reps/	2 sets, 8–12 reps/
2 sets, 8–12 reps/	2 sets, 8–12 reps/
2 sets, 8–12 reps/	2 sets, 8–12 reps/
1 set, 8–12 reps/	1 set, 8–12 reps/
1 set, 8–12 reps/	1 set, 8–12 reps/
2 sets, 8–12 reps/	2 sets, 8–12 reps/
2 sets, 8–12 reps/	2 sets, 8–12 reps/
2 sets, 8–12 reps/	2 sets, 8–12 reps/
2 sets, 10–15 reps/	2 sets, 10–15 reps/
2 sets, 10–15 reps/	2 sets, 10–15 reps/
2 sets, 10–15 reps/	2 sets, 10–15 reps/
1 set, 10–15 reps/	1 set, 10–15 reps/
1 set, 10–15 reps/	1 set, 10–15 reps/

(continued)

LEVEL-THREE EXERCISES, MONDAY AND FRIDAY	WEEK 1	
	WORKOUT 1	WORKOUT 2
Bench dip	2 sets, 8–12 reps/	2 sets, 8–12 reps/
Kickback	2 sets, 8–12 reps/	2 sets, 8–12 reps/
Overhead triceps extension	2 sets, 8–12 reps/	2 sets, 8–12 reps/
Zottman curl	2 sets, 8–12 reps/	2 sets, 8–12 reps/
Hammer curl	2 sets, 8–12 reps/	2 sets, 8–12 reps/
Biceps curl	2 sets, 8–12 reps/	2 sets, 8–12 reps/
Wrist curl	1 set, 8–12 reps/	1 set, 8–12 reps/
Reverse wrist curl	1 set, 8–12 reps/	1 set, 8–12 reps/
Squat	2 sets, 10–15 reps/	2 sets, 10–15 reps/
Lunge	2 sets, 10–15 reps/	2 sets, 10–15 reps/
Calf raise	2 sets, 10–15 reps/	2 sets, 10–15 reps/

LEVEL-THREE EXERCISES, WEDNESDAY	WORKOUT 1
Bench press	3 sets, 8–12 reps/
Bent-over row	3 sets, 8–12 reps/
Rotation press	3 sets, 8–12 reps/
Catch	3 sets, 8–12 reps/
Isometric back extension	3 sets, 4 reps (4 sec holds)/

velop any faster with additional exercises.

In Levels Two and Three you'll do other, new biceps and triceps exercises before repeating the ones you learned in Level One. So even though you'll do those same four Level-One exercises for 6 weeks, you'll do them with different levels of fatigue in each level. Your arm muscles will have to make continual physiological adjustments to the exercises, experiencing them somewhat differently in each of the three levels.

WEEK 2	
WORKOUT 1	**WORKOUT 2**
2 sets, 8–12 reps/	2 sets, 8–12 reps/
2 sets, 8–12 reps/	2 sets, 8–12 reps/
2 sets, 8–12 reps/	2 sets, 8–12 reps/
2 sets, 8–12 reps/	2 sets, 8–12 reps/
2 sets, 8–12 reps/	2 sets, 8–12 reps/
2 sets, 8–12 reps/	2 sets, 8–12 reps/
1 set, 8–12 reps/	1 set, 8–12 reps/
1 set, 8–12 reps/	1 set, 8–12 reps/
2 sets, 10–15 reps/	2 sets, 10–15 reps/
2 sets, 10–15 reps/	2 sets, 10–15 reps/
2 sets, 10–15 reps/	2 sets, 10–15 reps/
WORKOUT 1	
3 sets, 8–12 reps/	
3 sets, 8–12 reps/	
3 sets, 8–12 reps/	
3 sets, 8–12 reps/	
3 sets, 5 reps (4 sec holds)/	

SAFETY CONSIDERATIONS

Before beginning the Core Program, see a doctor if you're over 40 or have any special health concerns, such as high blood pressure, diabetes, heart problems, or obesity. Likewise, if you have orthopedic prob-lems—a bad back or a surgically repaired knee, for example—you should check in with your specialist before launching into this program. The Core Program is de-signed to be as safe and joint-friendly as a muscle-building workout can be, but your doctor may want you to modify the exercises in a way that the program doesn't anticipate.

That said, healthy guys shouldn't have any trouble with the Core Program. It's a versatile routine that should offer big benefits to guys of any age.

PERFORMANCE TIPS

To help you achieve proper form, each exercise in the Core Program is accompanied by performance tips that are specific to that particular exercise. Here's some general advice that applies to every exercise.

- Keep constant tension on your arms in every repetition of every set.
- Keep each motion slow and controlled, with no bouncing or jerking, for both the positive (lifting) and negative (lowering) phases of the exercise.
- Pause and flex your arm muscles at the top of the movement.
- Don't rest between repetitions—keep tension on your muscles and begin the next repetition immediately.
- Focus on feeling your arms doing the work. If you don't feel effort in your arms, you're wasting your time.
- Keep your lower back in its naturally arched position throughout each exercise. If you feel your back

muscles moving during an arm exercise, you're doing something wrong—using too much weight, perhaps, or continuing a set even though your arm muscles are thoroughly exhausted. Remember, when your form breaks down and you can no longer lift the weight using just your arm muscles, it's time to stop the set.

- Breathe on each repetition. Never hold your breath.

BEYOND THE EXERCISES

Each level of the Core Program includes a troubleshooting section that addresses problems and answers questions that beginning exercisers often encounter.

Additionally, all three levels present tips on achieving a better body through nutrition. The better you manage what goes into your stomach, the quicker you'll see muscle accumulate on your arms. And when you start putting on muscle through hard exercise and a solid diet, you start taking off fat. Plus, the smaller your waist is, the bigger your arms will look—a double benefit.

By the time you've completed the Core Program, you'll be well on the way to the fit, muscular body you want, with impressive arms and a shrinking waist. So what are you waiting for? Let's go for it.

CHAPTER NINE

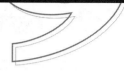

ESSENTIAL
BASICS
LEVEL ONE

In Level One of the Core Program, you'll learn the four fundamental exercises that will be the foundation of your entire 6-week arm-training routine, plus additional strength-training exercises to increase your production of muscle-building testosterone.

Here's the plan for Level One.

Do four arm exercises and five midsection and lower-body exercises twice a week.
Do three sessions of cardiovascular exercise.
Focus on getting enough protein to build muscle.

THE LEVEL-ONE ROUTINE

Do this routine two times a week, with at least 2 days' rest between workouts.
In Week 1, do one set of each exercise. In Week 2, do two sets of every exercise in the workout except the forearm exercises—stick to one set of each of them.
For the arm exercises, start with a weight you think you can lift for 8 repetitions. When you can do 12 repetitions with that weight, increase it.
For the lower-body exercises, start with a weight you think you can lift for 10 repetitions. When you can do 15, increase the weight.
Rest for 30 to 60 seconds between sets and exercises.

BENEFITS
OF LEVEL ONE

Stronger biceps and triceps

Higher energy levels

More strength and flexibility throughout your body

Release of muscle-building hormones through performance of lower-body strength exercises

Increased metabolism

Overhead Triceps Extension

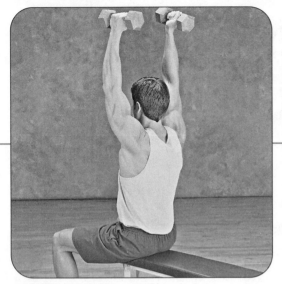

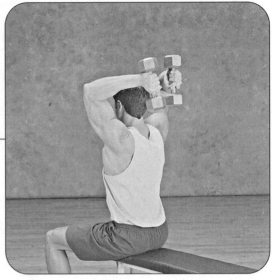

READY, SET:

Sit on a weight bench and hold a pair of dumbbells straight overhead. Your palms should face in toward each other, and your upper arms should be next to your ears.

GO:

Slowly bend your elbows to lower the weights behind you as far as you can without moving your upper arms.

Pause, then slowly lift the weights back to the starting position. Repeat.

PERFORMANCE TIPS

■ Your elbows should be your only moving parts. Keep your shoulders out of the movement by making sure your upper arms stay up next to your ears.

■ Keep your back in its natural alignment throughout the exercise.

■ Keep constant tension on your triceps. You want to feel the muscles stretching as you slowly lower the weights and contracting as you lift them.

Biceps Curl

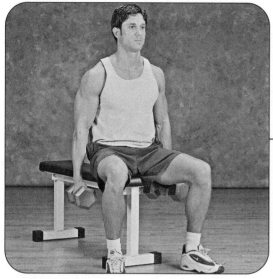

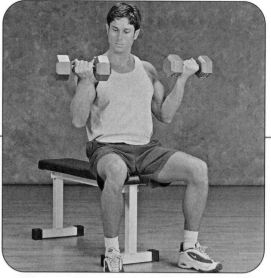

READY, SET:

Sit on the end of the bench and hold a pair of dumbbells with your arms hanging straight down from your shoulders.

GO:

Without moving your upper arms, bend your elbows to lift the weights toward your shoulders. As the weights move past your thighs, rotate your wrists upward (supinate) so your palms face your shoulders at the end of the movement. Stop when you've lifted the weights as high as you can without moving your upper arms.

Pause, then slowly lower the weights back to the starting position, rotating your wrists downward (pronating) until they're in the original position. Repeat.

PERFORMANCE TIPS

■ Keep your upper arms motionless and pressed against your sides throughout the movement. If you move your upper arms forward, you're using your shoulder muscles to help lift the weights.

■ Keep your back in its natural alignment throughout the exercise.

■ Use a full range of motion, but don't relax at the bottom of the movement. You want constant tension on your biceps through all parts of the repetition.

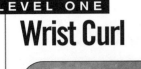

Wrist Curl

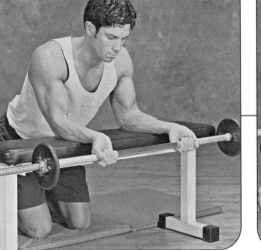

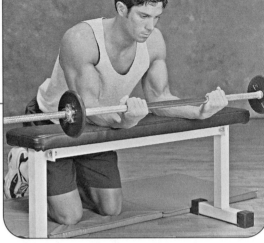

READY, SET:

Hold a barbell with an underhand, shoulder-width grip and kneel alongside the bench. Lay your forearms on the bench so your hands hang off the opposite side.

Without moving your forearms, bend your wrists to lower the weight toward the floor. Stop when you've lowered the weight as far as you can without moving your forearms.

GO:

Pause, then slowly lift the weight as high as you can toward your forearms. Pause again, slowly lower back to the starting position, and repeat.

PERFORMANCE TIPS

■ Keep your body in one position throughout the exercise; your wrists should be your only moving parts.

■ Don't let the barbell roll down into your fingers in the starting position. Having to roll it back up on each repetition burns out smaller muscles in your fingers and hands before you fully work the bigger muscles in your forearms.

■ You can also do this exercise with an EZ-curl bar (a cambered barbell) or dumbbells.

■ Another good variation is to hold the barbell behind your back, just below your buttocks, with your wrists facing away from you. It'll be a little harder to curl the weight from that position, because your forearms will be rotated and in a weaker position.

Reverse Wrist Curl

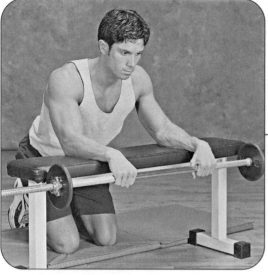
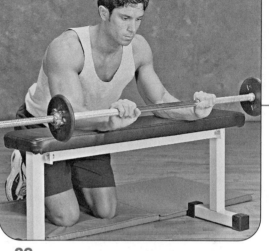

READY, SET:

Hold a barbell with an overhand, shoulder-width grip and kneel alongside the bench. Lay your forearms on the bench so your hands hang off the opposite side.

Without moving your forearms, bend your wrists to lower the weight toward the floor. Stop when you've lowered the weight as far as you can without moving your forearms.

GO:

Pause, then slowly lift the weight as high as you can toward your forearms. Pause again, slowly lower back to the starting position, and repeat.

PERFORMANCE TIPS

- Keep your body in one position throughout the exercise; your wrists should be your only moving parts.

- A good variation is to use dumbbells, sit on the bench, and position your forearms on your upper thighs with your hands hanging off your knees.

- Another joint-friendly variation is to use an EZ-curl bar. Hold the bar so your hands are at 45-degree angles.

Squat (Thighs and Gluteals)

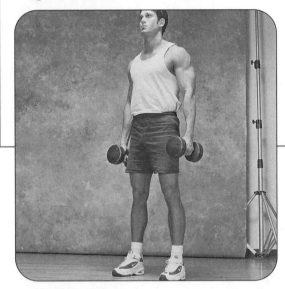 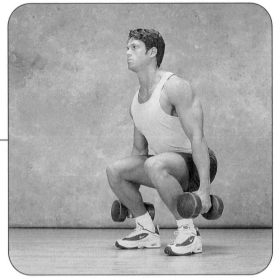

READY, SET:

Hold a pair of dumbbells and let your arms hang straight down from your shoulders. Stand with your feet about shoulder-width apart, your toes pointed slightly out, and your knees slightly bent. Pull your shoulders back, push your chest out, and look straight ahead. Your lower back should be neither arched nor rounded, and your head should be in alignment with your spine.

GO:

Bend your knees to lower yourself, and as you sink, sit back as if you were heading for a chair. Go down slowly until your thighs are parallel to the floor or until your heels start to rise off the floor.

Slowly rise back up to the starting position, and repeat.

PERFORMANCE TIPS

■ Try this without weights for your first workout. Hold your hands straight out from your shoulders.

■ Keep your heels flat on the floor and your back in its natural alignment. Try to descend until your upper thighs are parallel to the floor. It may take a while to get the hang of it, but when you do, you'll develop muscle fast.

■ Squats will make your knees stronger as long as you do them in a controlled fashion. Never lower yourself rapidly or bounce out of the bottom position—that is tough on your knees, and it doesn't do your lower back any favors.

Lunge (Thighs and Gluteals)

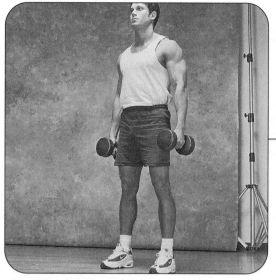

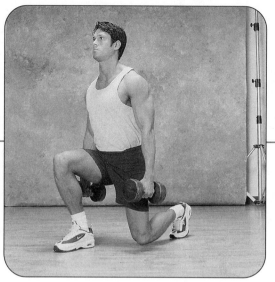

READY, SET:

Hold a pair of dumbbells and let your arms hang straight down from your shoulders. Stand with your feet a little wider than shoulder-width apart, your toes pointed slightly out, and your knees slightly bent. Pull your shoulders back, push your chest out, and look straight ahead. Your lower back should be neither arched nor rounded, and your head should be in alignment with your spine.

GO:

With your nondominant leg, step a little farther forward than you would in a normal stride, and land on your heel as you bend that knee 90 degrees and lower your other knee until it's just short of touching the floor.

Push back off your forward heel and return to the starting position. You can either finish all your reps with the same leg forward before switching to the other leg or alternate legs until you finish the set.

PERFORMANCE TIPS

■ Try this without weights for your first workout. When you can do 15 repetitions with each leg, add the dumbbells.

■ Start with your weaker leg, and always do the same number of repetitions with each leg. If you start with your stronger side, you may not be able to finish the same number with your weaker one, increasing your strength discrepancy.

■ Lengthen your stride until you can bend your forward knee 90 degrees and still keep it behind your toes. Never bounce your back knee off the ground.

■ Keep your torso upright. Don't let it drift forward as you get tired.

Calf Raise

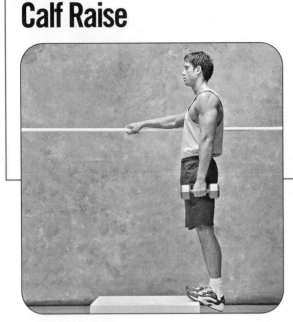
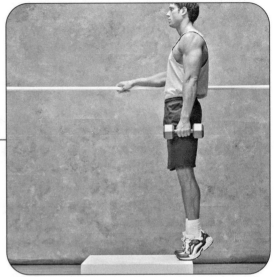

READY, SET:

Hold a dumbbell and let your arm hang straight down from your shoulder. Stand on the balls of your feet on a raised step or platform (a staircase works well) with your feet hip-width apart and your heels hanging off the step, as low as they'll go. Use your free hand to steady yourself.

GO:

Raise your heels as high as possible, distributing your weight toward your big toes.

Pause, then slowly return to the starting position. Pause again, and repeat.

PERFORMANCE TIPS

■ Each workout, alternate the hand in which you hold the weight. Or do half of the repetitions with the weight in one hand, then switch for the other half.

■ Always go as high as you can and as low as you can on each repetition, and pause for a full second in each position. You'll build the most muscle this way.

Crunch with a Cross (Abdominals)

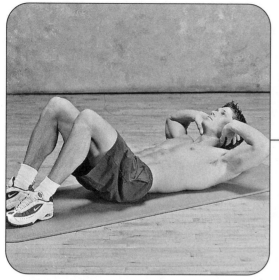 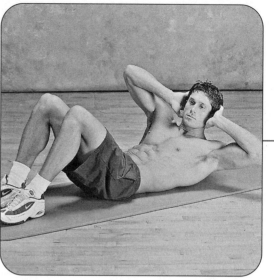

READY, SET:

Lie on your back with your knees bent, your feet flat on the floor, your head and neck relaxed, and your hands behind your ears.

GO:

Use your upper abs to raise your rib cage toward your pelvis and lift your shoulder blades off the floor as you cross your right shoulder toward your left knee.

Pause, then slowly lower back to the starting position. Repeat, this time crossing your left shoulder toward your right knee. That's one repetition.

PERFORMANCE TIPS

- Make sure your shoulder blades come off the floor each time. Don't just move your head and neck.
- Raise and lower yourself slowly; don't use momentum to get through the repetitions.
- Keep constant tension on your abs throughout the movement—don't rest at the bottom of the movement.
- Pause at the top of the movement, after you've exhaled, and feel the squeeze go deeper into your abdominals.
- Keep your head and neck relaxed.

Opposite Arm and Leg Raise (Lower Back)

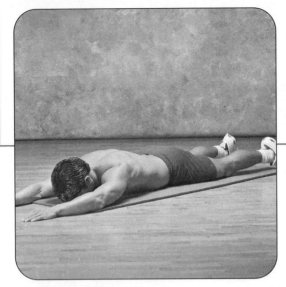 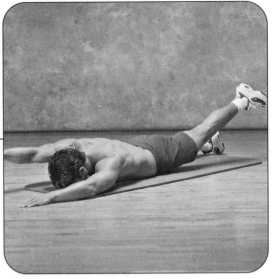

READY, SET:

Lie facedown on the floor with your arms and legs extended. Your palms should face the floor.

GO:

Simultaneously raise your right arm and left leg to a comfortable height.

Hold for 2 seconds, then slowly lower to the starting position. As soon as your arm and leg lightly touch the floor, repeat with your left arm and right leg. Alternate until you've done all the recommended repetitions on each side.

PERFORMANCE TIPS

■ As you raise your arm and leg, also try to extend them—that is, make them reach out farther.

■ As you raise your leg, you'll feel this exercise in your gluteals and hamstrings as well as in your lower back.

■ If it feels too easy to simply raise one arm and leg, try keeping your nonworking arm and leg off the floor throughout the exercise. So while you raise your right arm and left leg, keep your left arm and right leg off the floor slightly. Then, as you lift the latter limbs, stop short of touching your right arm and left leg to the floor. That will keep more tension on your lower back throughout the set.

■ My lower back hurts when I do the arm exercises.

If the pain shoots into other areas, such as your legs and neck, or becomes so severe that you can't do normal daily activities after working out, go to a doctor and get checked out. Here are some suggestions for preventing less serious pain.

1. Make sure you're thoroughly warmed up before lifting. If the recommended 5-minute warmup doesn't seem to be enough, increase it to 10 minutes.

2. Double up on the lower-back stretches in chapter 5. Do each twice. But don't try to stretch past the point of pain. Make these gentle, slow stretches, allowing your back to relax rather than tighten out of fear that you're going to do some serious damage.

3. When you're lifting, keep your hips in their natural, neutral position. Don't allow them to tilt forward or back. A good way to make sure that you're positioned correctly is to sit sideways to a mirror and watch your posture as you lift.

4. Relax your jaw. It sounds weird, but some guys clench their jaws when they lift, and this can create problems elsewhere. Try to keep your mouth slightly open throughout the exercises. This technique will also remind you to breathe on each repetition.

■ I don't know if I'm using enough weight.

Let the repetitions be your guide. The perfect weight for the Core Program arm exercises is one that allows you to do 8 repetitions with good form. But it's rare that you'll hit exactly 8. More likely, you'll do 9 or 10, which is fine. Then, if you manage 12 the next workout, you know you need to increase. Conversely, if you can't do more than 5 with good form, you've chosen a weight that's too heavy.

■ I don't feel these exercises in my arms.

It takes time to get used to the way your muscles feel when they're exercising. Rest assured, you'll soon notice every little nuance of every new exercise you try.

That said, arm exercises are usually the easiest to feel. In fact, many guys think they're working their arms even when they're not. The problem, most likely, is that you're cheating by using the wrong muscles to lift the weight.

When you do a biceps curl, you're cheating if you shrug your shoulders and push up on your toes to get the weights moving, then bend backward to complete the repetition. The correct way to do this exercise is to start with your shoulders and lower body in a set position and try not to move them at all during the exercise.

Cheating during a triceps extension is pushing off with your legs to get the weights moving, or dropping your elbows down in front of your face. In the latter case, you're shifting the weights so they're not moving against gravity. To do the extension fair and square, keep your upper arms perpendicular to the floor, with your elbows pointed toward the ceiling. That way, the weights are always moving against the full force of gravity.

Finally, make sure you use enough weight. The last repetition of each set should require the absolute last bit of effort that your arm muscles can muster.

AEROBIC ESSENTIALS:
YOUR CARDIO CALENDAR

As discussed in chapter 3, you should ideally do a half-hour of aerobic exercise three times a week, with 20 minutes of that in your target heart-rate zone (65 to 85 percent of your maxinum heart rate—your max is 220 minus your age).

That could be a little too much if you're a complete beginner to exercise. In that case, do the following three times a week.

■ 5 minutes at easy pace
■ 5 minutes at target pace
■ 5 minutes at easy pace

If you're already in decent shape, do the full prescription.

■ 5 minutes at easy pace
■ 20 minutes at target pace
■ 5 minutes at easy pace

If possible, do these workouts on days when you don't lift.

When it's impossible to exercise that many days a week and you need to do aerobics on the same day you lift, do the cardio after the weights. If you do cardio first, you'll burn off some of the muscle fuel you need to give a full effort in the weight room. To get bigger muscles, you have to lift when you're fresh. Don't worry; you'll have plenty of energy left for aerobics.

Another benefit to doing aerobics last is that you'll use more fat calories after you've already expended muscle fuel by lifting weights. The impact isn't huge, but over the course of a year you could burn off an extra pound or two of fat.

EATING ESSENTIALS:
PROTEIN POWER

The Core Program recommendation is 7 to 10 grams of protein for every 10 pounds of body weight every day. The top end of that range is a little beyond what science has shown to be the maximum amount of protein a body can use, but it's an easy figure to remember.

Most of that protein should come from lean meats, fish, eggs, beans, and low-fat dairy products. You'll also pick up some from nuts, bread, pasta, and rice.

TO SUPPLEMENT
OR NOT TO SUPPLEMENT

When you look at the foods you have to buy or prepare daily to get the protein needed for best muscle building, you understand why the supplement industry exists.

A meal-replacement shake can be ready in a minute—you just throw the powder into a blender or shaker cup, add water, mix, and drink. For this minimal effort, you get about 40 grams of protein in a 300-calorie shake that may actually taste decent. What's more, the protein in the meal replacements, usually whey or a blend of whey and casein, has what scientists call high bioavailability—that is, your body can easily use it to build muscle.

What often stops people from taking advantage of these supplements is the price. A box of 20 packets of a popular meal replacement like Myoplex, MetRx, or Grow! usually costs around $35. That's less than $2 per shake, but it adds up over the course of a month.

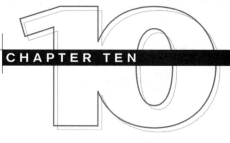

CHAPTER TEN

ESSENTIAL
BUILDUP
LEVEL TWO

Ready to learn new moves and add new challenges? Here's your workout for Level Two.

Increase your arm workout to six exercises.

Add three upper-body exercises to work your chest, back, and shoulders.

Increase your aerobic workouts, if you're a beginner, to 24 minutes in Week 1 of Level Two, then to 28 minutes in Week 2. If you're more advanced, switch one aerobic session to an interval workout.

Get the right mix of nutrients before your workout to give you enough energy to lift weights intensely, and eat the right stuff after that workout to help you recover.

THE LEVEL-TWO ROUTINE

Perform the total-body workout two times a week.

In Week 1, do one set of each exercise. In Week 2, do two sets of every exercise in the workout except the forearm, abdominal, and lower-back exercises—stick to one set of each of them.

Do 8 to 12 repetitions of each upper-body exercise, including the arm exercises, and 10 to 15 repetitions of the lower-body exercises.

Rest for 30 to 60 seconds between sets and exercises.

BENEFITS
OF LEVEL TWO

Increased strength and endurance in your arms

Improved aerobic capacity

Weight loss from increased exercise

Smaller waistline from a speeded-up metabolism

More energy from your higher fitness level and careful attention to pre- and postworkout nutrition

More head-to-toe strength and muscular endurance from the full-body workout

Kickback

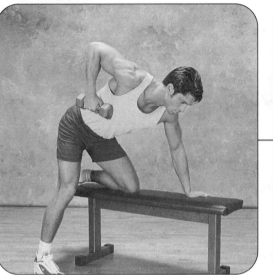
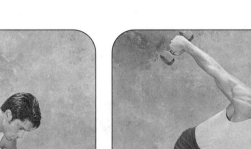

READY, SET:

Hold a dumbbell with your nondominant hand, palm facing in. Put your opposite hand and knee on the bench so that your upper body is at about a 90-degree angle. Your back should be flat and parallel to the bench and the floor. Raise the dumbbell straight up to the side of your abdomen, and point your elbow up toward the ceiling.

GO:

Keeping your elbow pointing straight up, slowly straighten your arm, lifting the weight as high as you can toward the ceiling.

Pause, then slowly lower the weight back to the starting position. Repeat. When you finish all of your repetitions with your nondominant arm, hold the weight in your dominant hand and do the same number of reps with that arm.

PERFORMANCE TIPS

■ Most people do this exercise with their upper arms parallel to the floor. If you do that, your triceps have to work in only the last couple of inches of your range of motion; there's no resistance from gravity until you get to that point. Raise your upper arm as high as possible so you fight gravity all the way up.

■ Keep your torso fixed in one place. If you move it, you add momentum to the exercise, taking work away from your triceps.

Overhead Triceps Extension

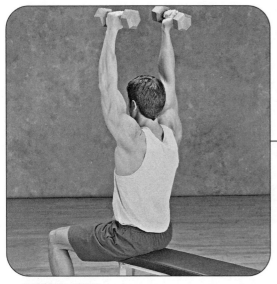 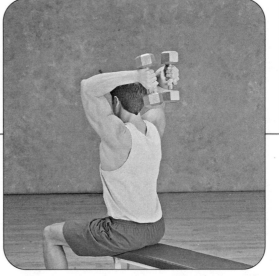

READY, SET:

Sit on the bench and hold a pair of dumbbells straight overhead. Your palms should face in toward each other, and your upper arms should be next to your ears.

GO:

Slowly bend your elbows to lower the weights behind you as far as you can without moving your upper arms.

Pause, then slowly lift the weights back to the starting position. Repeat.

PERFORMANCE TIPS

■ Your elbows should be your only moving parts. Keep your shoulders out of the movement by making sure your upper arms stay up next to your ears.

■ Keep your back in its natural alignment throughout the exercise.

■ Keep constant tension on your triceps. You want to feel the muscles stretching as you slowly lower the weights and contracting as you lift them.

Hammer Curl

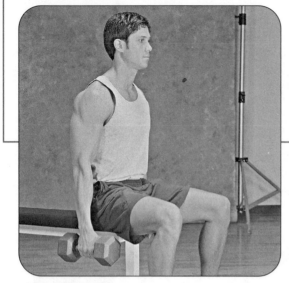

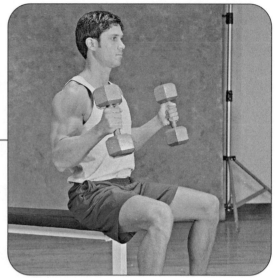

READY, SET:

Sit on the end of the bench and hold a pair of dumb-bells with your arms hanging straight down from your shoulders.

GO:

Without moving your upper arms, bend your elbows to lift the weights toward your shoulders, keeping your palms facing inward. Stop when you've lifted the weights as high as you can without moving your upper arms.

Pause, then slowly lower the weights back to the starting position. Repeat.

PERFORMANCE TIPS

■ Keep your upper arms pressed against your sides throughout the exercise.

■ Keep your back in its natural alignment throughout the exercise.

■ Don't rest at the bottom of the movement; keep constant tension on your arms.

Biceps Curl

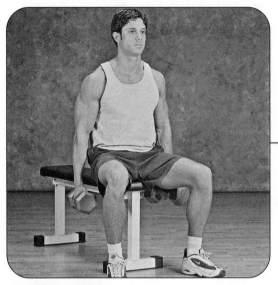 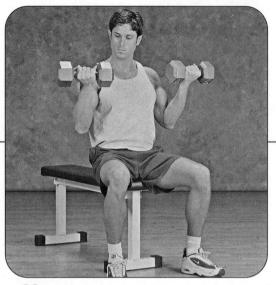

READY, SET:

Sit on the end of the bench and hold a pair of dumbbells with your arms hanging straight down from your shoulders.

GO:

Without moving your upper arms, bend your elbows to lift the weights toward your shoulders. As the weights move past your thighs, rotate your wrists upward (supinate) so your palms face your shoulders at the end of the movement. Stop when you've lifted the weights as high as you can without moving your upper arms.

Pause, then slowly lower the weights back to the starting position, rotating your wrists downward (pronating) until they're in the original position. Repeat.

PERFORMANCE TIPS

- Keep your upper arms motionless and pressed against your sides throughout the movement. If you move your upper arms forward, you're using your shoulder muscles to help lift the weights.

- Keep your back in its natural alignment throughout the exercise.

- Use a full range of motion, but don't relax at the bottom of the movement. You want constant tension on your biceps through all parts of the repetition.

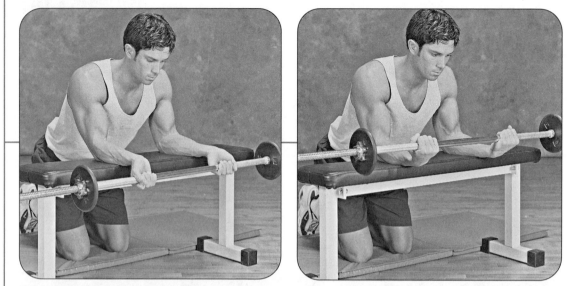

WRIST CURL: Hold the barbell with an underhand grip, and bend your wrists to lower it toward the floor. Then slowly lift the weight as high as you can toward your forearms.

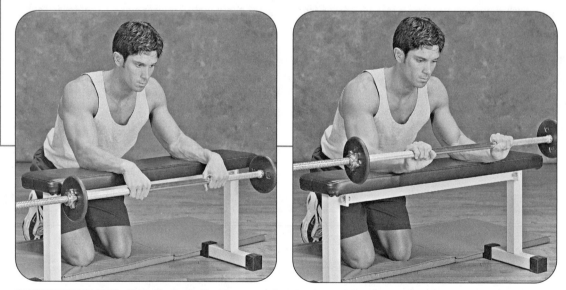

REVERSE WRIST CURL: Hold the barbell with an overhand grip, and bend your wrists to lower it toward the floor. Then slowly lift the weight as high as you can toward your forearms.

▲ *If you need a refresher on the specific instructions for these exercises, see pages 60 and 61.*

Bench Press (Chest, Triceps, and Shoulders)

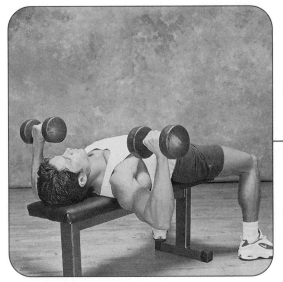

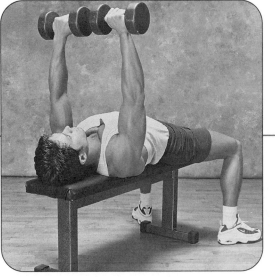

READY, SET:

Grab a pair of dumbbells in an overhand grip. Lie on the bench with your feet flat on the floor for stability. Hold the weights just above and outside your chest.

GO:

Push the weights up in a slanting motion so they almost meet when your arms are fully extended.

Slowly lower back to the starting position, pause, and repeat.

PERFORMANCE TIPS

■ Most guys who haven't lifted before have a strength discrepancy, meaning that one arm is stronger than the other, especially if they play sports that use one arm more than the other. So it may be tough at first to get both dumbbells moving at the same speed and in the same range of motion. Once you get the coordination down, your strength will increase rapidly—and evenly.

■ Keep your lower back in its natural position throughout the exercise. Don't allow it to arch excessively so you can push up heavier weights.

■ Don't clank the weights together at the top. It takes tension off your muscles.

■ Lower the weights as far as they want to go—that's your natural range of motion on this exercise. If you try to stop them short of a full descent or lower them past your comfort zone, you risk straining your shoulders and limiting your gains.

Bent-Over Row (Upper Back and Biceps)

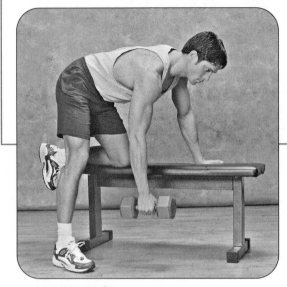
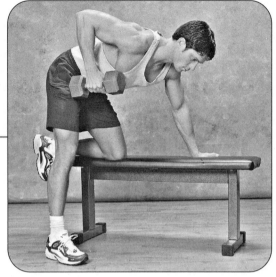

READY, SET:

Hold a dumbbell with your nondominant hand, palm facing in. Put your opposite hand and knee on a weight bench so that your upper body is at about a 90-degree angle. Your back should be flat and parallel to the bench and the floor. Let your nondominant arm hang straight down from your shoulder. Tighten your abs for stability.

GO:

Pull the weight straight up toward the side of your abdomen, and point your elbow up toward the ceiling.

Pause, then slowly lower the weight back to the starting position. Repeat.

When you finish all of your repetitions with your nondominant arm, hold the weight in your dominant hand and do the same number of reps with that arm.

PERFORMANCE TIPS

■ Focus on your back muscles: Think of them pulling your arm back to start the movement, rather than starting the movement with your arm.

■ Keep your torso in one fixed position throughout the exercise. If you add any body rotation to the movement, you take your back muscles out of the exercise.

■ Momentum is the enemy. That's why you should pause at the top and bottom of the movement. If you do that and lower the weight slowly, you'll work your back muscles on the way up and the way down.

Rotation Press (Shoulders and Triceps)

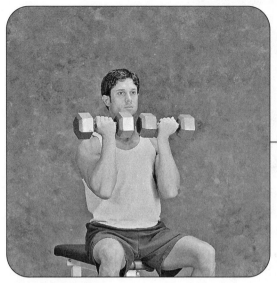 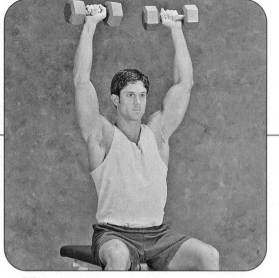

READY, SET:

Sit on the end of the bench and hold a pair of dumbbells underneath your chin with your hands rotated so the backs face forward. Pull your shoulders back, push your chest out, and look straight ahead.

GO:

Push the weights up directly over your head, rotating your hands so your palms face forward when your arms are fully extended.

Pause, then slowly lower the weights back to the starting position, rotating your hands back again. Repeat.

PERFORMANCE TIPS

■ Keep your torso in the same position throughout the lift. Don't allow yourself to lean back as you push the weights over your head—that's murder on your lower back.

■ Don't bring the dumbbells together at the top; your shoulders will work harder if you keep the weights apart.

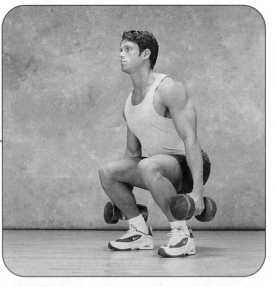

SQUAT: Bend your knees to lower yourself until your thighs are parallel to the floor or until your heels start to rise off the floor, slowly rise back up.

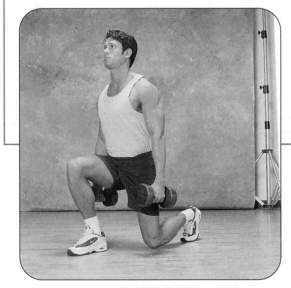

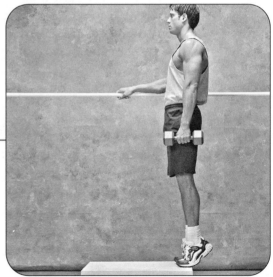

LUNGE: Step forward and bend your knee while lowering your other knee toward the floor, then rise.

CALF RAISE: Raise your heels as high as possible, then slowly lower.

▲ *If you need a refresher on the specific instructions for these exercises, see pages 62, 63, and 64.*

Crossover (Abdominals)

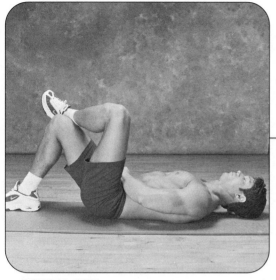

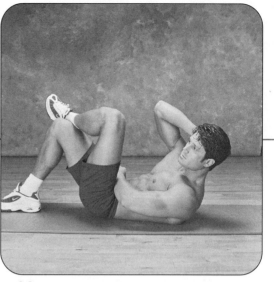

READY, SET:

Lie on your back with your knees up and your feet on the floor. Cross your left leg over your right leg. Your left ankle should rest just below your right knee, making a triangle between your legs. Put your right hand behind your head, with your elbow extended to the side. Rest your head and elbow on the floor. Place your left hand on your right obliques or at your left side.

GO:

Use your right obliques to raise your right shoulder and cross it toward your left knee.

Then slowly lower your shoulder back to the starting position. As soon as your shoulder blade lightly touches the floor, repeat.

When you finish all of your repetitions on your right side, switch positions to work your left side: Put your right ankle below your left knee, put your left hand behind your head, and raise your left shoulder toward your right knee. Do the same number of reps on your left side.

PERFORMANCE TIPS

■ Feel the squeeze in your oblique muscles on the side that you're working. You'll probably also feel it in your upper abs on that side, which is fine.

■ Don't rest at the bottom of the movement; keep constant tension on your abs.

■ Move up and down slowly; don't use momentum to finish your repetitions.

Superman (Lower Back)

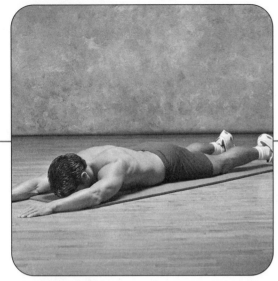 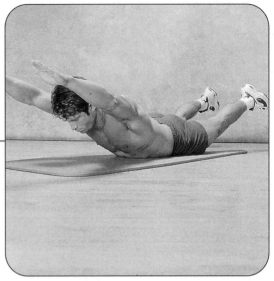

READY, SET:

Lie facedown on the floor with your arms and legs extended and angled out slightly. Your palms should face the floor.

GO:

Lift your arms and legs off the floor as if you were Superman flying. Hold for 3 seconds.

Then slowly lower your arms and legs back to the starting position. As they lightly touch the floor, repeat.

PERFORMANCE TIPS

■ Your head and neck will also rise off the floor on this exercise, but don't allow your neck to hyperextend backward. Keep your neck in line with your shoulders throughout the exercise. However much your shoulders rise, that's how high your neck should lift.

■ As in the lower-back exercise in Level One (the opposite arm and leg raise), you'll feel a contraction in your gluteals and hamstrings too.

■ If you can hold each contraction for longer than 3 seconds, do so. The more endurance you build in your lower back, the more improvements you'll feel in your posture.

INCREASE YOUR INTENSITY

The traditional prescription for getting better results from aerobic exercise is to do your workout for a longer length of time. If you're a beginning exerciser, this approach is appropriate. You still need to work toward your goal of 20 minutes in your target heart-rate zone, three times a week.

The Beginner Plan

On 3 nonconsecutive days in Week 1 of Level Two, do this 24-minute aerobic workout.

5 minutes at easy pace
6 minutes at target pace
2 minutes at easy pace
6 minutes at target pace
5 minutes at easy pace

In Week 2 of Level Two, increase to a 28-minute workout on each of your three aerobic days.

5 minutes at easy pace
8 minutes at target pace
2 minutes at easy pace
8 minutes at target pace
5 minutes at easy pace

But when you're trying to build muscle, you should keep the length of your workout the same and instead crank up the intensity. So if you can easily handle the 20 minutes in your target heart-rate zone that were prescribed in Level One, you should now do an interval workout in place of one of your aerobic workouts.

The Advanced Plan

In one of your three aerobics sessions, try this interval workout.

■ 5 minutes at easy pace
■ 30 seconds at hard pace—not all-out like a sprint but the best effort you can put out for 30 seconds
■ 1 minute at easy pace (Just take a brisk walk or light jog if you're running, or drop a couple of levels on a cardio machine)
■ Repeat for a total of 8 to 12 30-second intervals and 1-minute recovery periods
■ 5 minutes at easy pace for a cooldown (The 1 minute at easy pace during your final interval can count as part of this cooldown)

You can do these intervals on any aerobic machine in the gym or while running, cycling, swimming, inline skating—pretty much any aerobic activity you can think of.

PRE- AND POSTWORKOUT FEEDING

The longer you stick with an exercise program, the more you notice how different one workout can be from the next. Some days, you're a superhero, effortlessly flinging about weights of immense proportions; other days, you're a feeble, old geezer who can barely lift himself up out of the recliner.

Any number of factors could cause you to have a lousy workout when you think you're due for a great one. You could be coming down with an illness or under too

■ Why don't I see any changes in my arms yet?
If you're new to weight lifting, it takes a few weeks to see muscle growth, and there's nothing you can do to speed up that process.

If you were working out regularly before you started the Core Program but you still don't see results yet, you could have some fat in your arms that's preventing you from seeing the peak in your biceps and the developing horseshoe in your triceps. Diligent attention to your diet and full intensity in your workouts will steadily whittle that fat away.

If there's no fat in your arms, you may not be eating enough to make your muscles grow. Try adding a little food to each meal: an extra glass of milk, one more piece of whole-wheat toast, a container of low-fat yogurt. Don't add more than 500 calories a day to your diet. That could cause your body to store the excess as fat instead of muscle. But muscles can't be made of air—you have to give them sufficient food to help them grow.

■ Level Two has six arm exercises and eight exercises for other muscle groups. Shouldn't those numbers be reversed: eight exercises for my arms and six for everything else?
By the 4th week of the Core Program, you're doing two sets of two exercises for both your biceps and triceps (not counting your forearm exercises). That's plenty of growth stimulus for such small, simple muscles. Put your best effort into those four sets for biceps and four sets for triceps, and you'll see results. (If you don't put in full effort, it doesn't matter how many sets and exercises you do. Mediocre effort yields mediocre results.)

You're also doing two sets of bench presses and two of rotation presses, which work your triceps along with your chest and shoulders, plus two sets of bent-over rows, which work your biceps along with your back. That's a total of eight sets working your triceps and six exerting your biceps. (Don't worry about creating an imbalance between those muscles; your triceps have almost twice as much muscle mass as your biceps do, so if you want extra upper-arm beef, there's more room to add it in your triceps.)

And remember what you learned in chapter 2: Big-muscle exercises like squats, lunges, presses, and rows stimulate the most testosterone, your body's number one muscle-building hormone. Arm exercises don't provoke that same response from your hormonal system.

■ I'm suddenly less adept at the arm exercises from Level One. How come I can't do those as well as I did them a week ago?
You're doing new exercises before the old ones, so your arms are dealing with a new level of exhaustion. That's part of the plan. Once you learn to do an exercise, the next thing to do is make it more difficult so your arm muscles have to learn to do it again, this time while exhausted. This variety is what provokes your body to make rapid adaptations. At first, those adaptations are neurological: Your body learns to recruit more muscle fibers and nerve cells to make your arm muscles stronger. But eventually, you run out of new fibers and nerves to bring into the exercises, and your body starts making the muscle cells larger.

much stress at work or home, for example. But there's also a good chance that you haven't timed your meals properly.

Hunger pangs can take your mind off your workout, leaving one thought in your head: "Must . . . eat . . . now!" On the other hand, one of the most unpleasant feelings you can have while exercising is a churning stomach in which an undigested meal is tossed about by waves of digestive juices. Here's how to avoid these distractions and make sure you take in just the right amount of grub.

PREWORKOUT MEAL

Try to eat an hour or two before your workout. If you know you're going to work out at 5:30 in the evening, for example, make sure you eat something between 3:30 and 4:30 in the afternoon. That should give you the energy to exercise without causing the sluggishness that comes from eating too close to a workout. The bigger the meal, the more time you want to put between it and your workout.

What to eat: Fat and fiber take the longest to empty from your stomach, so avoid those in the last 2 hours before a workout. That leaves protein and nonfibrous carbohydrates. For an ideal preexercise meal, get out your blender and throw in 1 cup of grape juice, 1 cup of fat-free milk, 1 cup of fat-free plain yogurt, 1 cup of fresh or frozen strawberries, and, if you want, 1 scoop of whey protein powder. Add a few ice cubes if you're using fresh fruit instead of frozen. Blend until smooth. And skip the fruit if you're

within an hour of your workout—the fiber will speed up the digestive process.

POSTWORKOUT MEAL

Most guys think that they need protein, protein, and more protein after a workout. But studies show that carbohydrates are actually the most important nutrient following exercise. Carbohydrates stimulate insulin production, and insulin is the rapid-transit system that gets nutrients to your muscles to refuel and repair them.

What to eat: This is the one time in your day when you should eat fast-acting carbohydrates like white bread, instant rice, or baked potatoes. Those provoke the greatest and fastest surge of insulin. Another option is to use a meal-replacement powder that includes a fast-moving protein like maltodextrin.

Or have a carbs-rich shake immediately after your workout and a meal an hour or two later. For the shake, combine 1 cup of orange juice, 1 cup of fat-free milk, 1 of cup fat-free vanilla yogurt, a banana, and 1 cup of fresh or frozen unsweetened blueberries in your blender (which you washed all the dried-on strawberry gunk off of, right?). Add a handful of ice cubes if the blueberries are fresh. Blend until smooth.

Your meal should include protein, carbohydrates, and healthy fat like that found in olive oil. Try a baked or grilled chicken breast, a baked potato with fat-free sour cream, and a mixed-green salad with olive oil–based dressing. You can even have a scoop of ice cream for dessert.

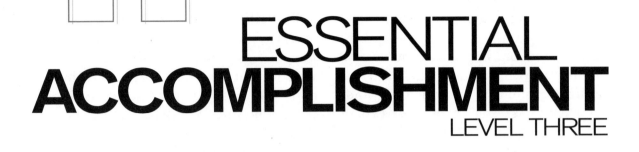

CHAPTER ELEVEN

ESSENTIAL
ACCOMPLISHMENT
LEVEL THREE

In the next 2 weeks, you have your work cut out for you. It'll be worth it, though, when your arms are cut out too.

■ Perform two new exercises for your arms.
■ If you're a beginner, increase your aerobic exercise to 30 minutes, three times a week, including 20 minutes in your target heart-rate zone. If you're more advanced, substitute a sprint workout for one of your aerobic workouts.
■ Adjust the fat and carbohydrates in your diet.

THE LEVEL-THREE ROUTINE

■ Focus on your arms and legs on Monday and Friday, and work your chest, back, shoulders, and midsection on Wednesday.
■ In the arm-and-leg workout, do two sets of each exercise except the forearm exercises—stick to one set of each of them.
■ In the other workout, do three sets of each exercise.
■ Do 8 to 12 repetitions of each upper-body exercise. Do 10 to 15 reps of each lower-body exercise except the isometric back extension—see the "Performance Tips" for that one. Once you hit the top end of the range with any weight on any exercise, increase the weight the next time you do that exercise.
■ Rest for 30 to 60 seconds between sets and exercises.

BENEFITS
OF LEVEL THREE

A tremendous muscle-building stimulus for your arms

Increased efficiency of your heart and lungs from aerobic exercise

Accelerated fat loss from the higher volume of exercise

Bench Dip

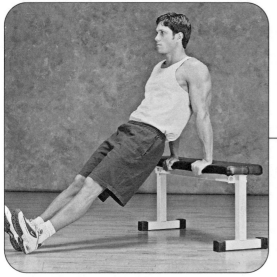

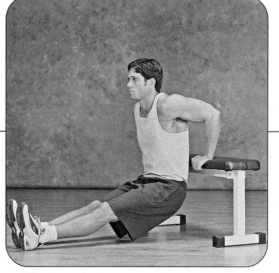

READY, SET:

Sit on the side of a weight bench. Place your palms, fingers forward, on the bench beside your hips. Push up with both arms until they are fully extended, and move your torso forward so that your butt and back are just in front of the bench.

GO:

Bend your elbows to a 90-degree angle, lowering your butt toward the floor.

Pause, then slowly raise back up to the starting position. Repeat.

PERFORMANCE TIPS

■ Maintain a flat back and raised chest throughout the exercise.

■ Move in a strict vertical line. Don't let your hips slide forward.

■ Keep your forearms vertical throughout the exercise.

■ Don't bounce at the bottom of the movement.

■ You can make this exercise more challenging in a variety of ways: Extend your legs until they're straight, place both legs on a second bench in front of you, place weight plates on your lap, or have a partner press down on your shoulders as you raise back up.

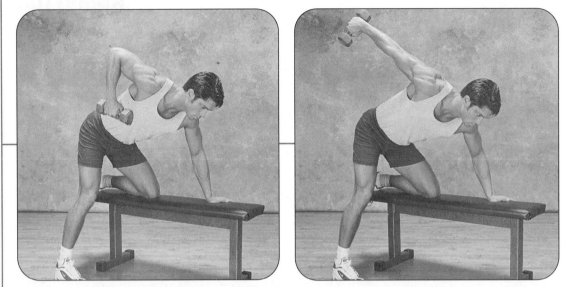

KICKBACK: Raise the dumbbell to the side of your abdomen, and point your elbow toward the ceiling. Keeping your elbow pointing up, lift the weight as high as you can toward the ceiling, then lower.

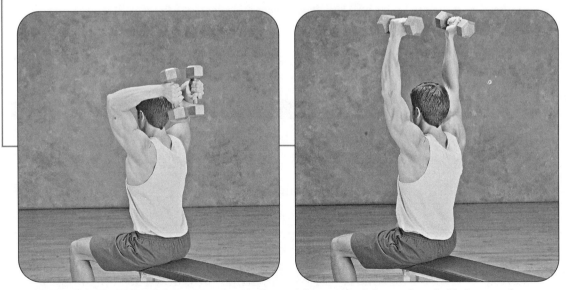

OVERHEAD TRICEPS EXTENSION: Hold the dumbbells straight overhead, lower them behind you as far as you can, then lift them back up.

▲ *If you need a refresher on the specific instructions for these exercises, see pages 70 and 71.*

Zottman Curl

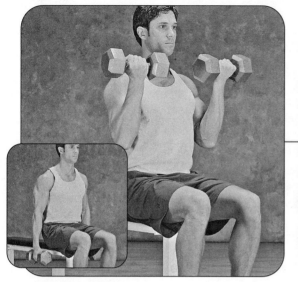

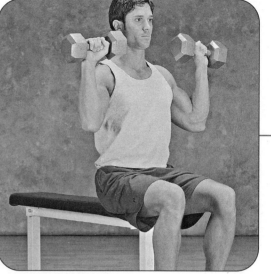

READY, SET:

Sit on the end of the bench and hold a pair of dumb-bells with your arms hanging straight down from your shoulders.

GO:

Without moving your upper arms, bend your elbows to lift the weights toward your shoulders while ro-tating your wrists upward (supinating) so your palms face your shoulders at the end of the movement.

KEEP GOING . . .

When you can't raise the weights any higher without allowing your upper arms to move forward, pause, then rotate your wrists downward (pronate).

Slowly lower the weights back to the starting po-sition, rotating your wrists back to the original po-sition at the end. Repeat.

PERFORMANCE TIPS

- Keep your upper arms pressed against your sides throughout the exercise.

- The Zottman Curl can also be performed while standing, including while standing with your back against a wall. You may also use a synchronized movement, raising one dumbbell while lowering the other. Or you may prefer to work one arm at a time: Perform the prescribed number of repetitions with your nondominant arm and then work the other.

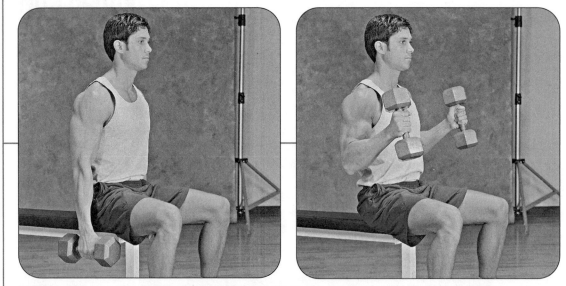

HAMMER CURL: Hold the dumbbells straight down, lift them toward your shoulders, then lower.

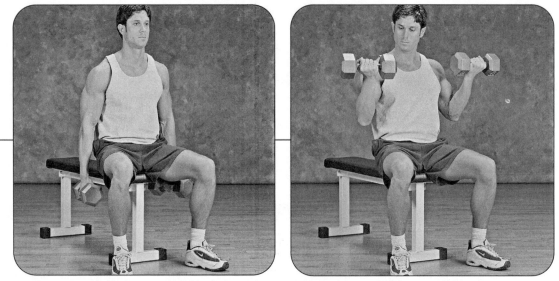

BICEPS CURL: Hold the dumbbells straight down, lift them toward your shoulders while rotating your wrists upward (supinating), then lower, rotating your wrists downward (pronating).

▲ *If you need a refresher on the specific instructions for these exercises, see pages 72 and 73.*

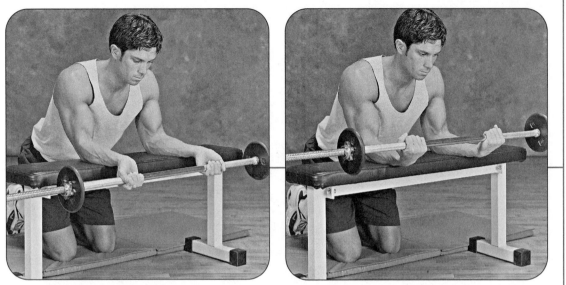

WRIST CURL: Hold the barbell with an underhand grip, and bend your wrists to lower it toward the floor. Then slowly lift the weight as high as you can toward your forearms.

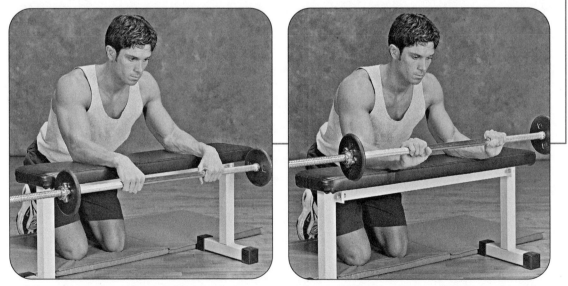

REVERSE WRIST CURL: Hold the barbell with an overhand grip, and bend your wrists to lower it toward the floor. Then slowly lift the weight as high as you can toward your forearms.

▲ *If you need a refresher on the specific instructions for these exercises, see pages 60 and 61.*

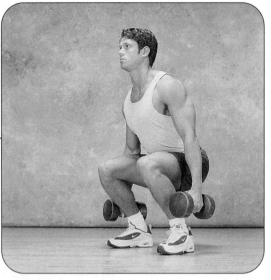

SQUAT: If you weren't able to get your upper thighs parallel to the floor in Level Two, try to descend a little lower this time. The longer your range of motion, the more strength and muscle you'll develop.

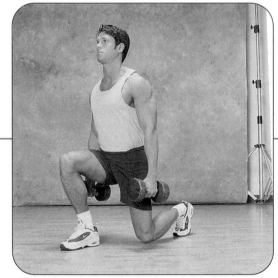

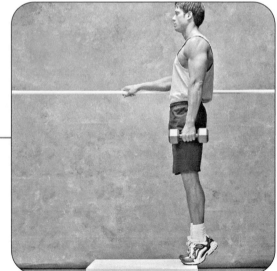

LUNGE: If you find the dumbbells awkward or struggle to maintain your grip, try the lunge with a barbell across your shoulders. The rest of the exercise is the same.

CALF RAISE: If you would rather work one calf at a time instead of doing the exercise as shown here, tuck the nonworking foot behind your working calf, and hold the weight on the side you're working.

▲ *If you need a refresher on the specific instructions for these exercises, see pages 62, 63, and 64.*

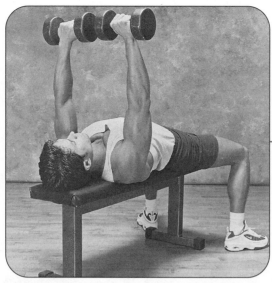

BENCH PRESS: Raise the dumbbells so they almost meet, then lower. A pushup works the same muscles as a bench press, so if you want extra work for your chest, you can add a set of pushups right after your presses. Do as many as you can.

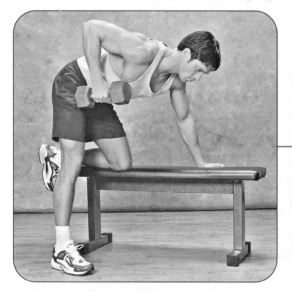

BENT-OVER ROW: Raise the dumbbell to the side of your abdomen, point your elbow toward the ceiling, then lower.

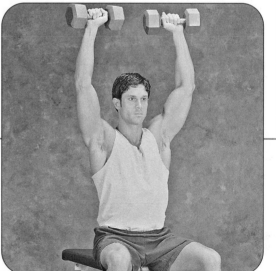

ROTATION PRESS: Raise the dumbbells over your head, rotating your hands so your palms face forward, then lower, rotating your hands back again.

▲ *If you need a refresher on the specific instructions for these exercises, see pages 75, 76, and 77.*

Catch (Abdominals)

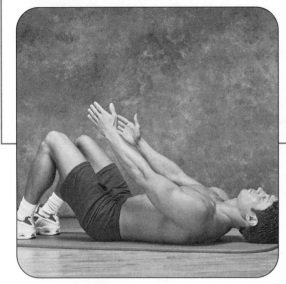 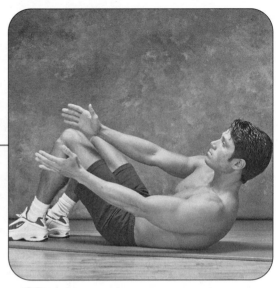

READY, SET:

Lie on your back with your knees bent, your feet flat on the floor, and your hands extended toward your knees.

GO:

Use your ab muscles to raise your torso on a diagonal line, lifting your right shoulder toward your left knee and reaching both hands above and to the outside of your left knee as if you were going to catch a ball that was being thrown to you. Hold for a second.

Then, in a controlled motion, slowly lower your shoulder back to the starting position. As soon as your shoulder blade lightly touches the floor, do the movement to your right side, lifting your left shoulder toward your right knee. That's one repetition.

PERFORMANCE TIPS

■ With your head completely unsupported, you may feel a little discomfort in your neck. You can try supporting it with one hand and reaching with the other hand.

Isometric Back Extension (Lower Back)

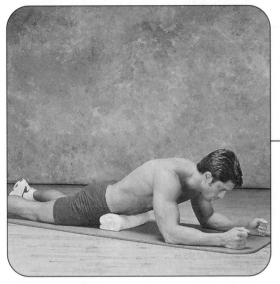

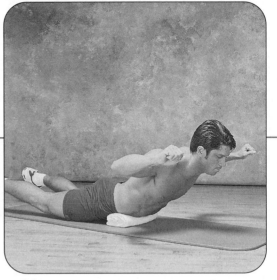

READY, SET:

Lie facedown on the floor with a rolled-up towel beneath your navel and your legs about shoulder-width apart. Lift your torso and rest your weight on your forearms, as if you were lying on the floor to watch TV.

GO:

Slowly lift your forearms off the floor and out to your sides while keeping your torso in the same position. Hold for the count specified in the "Performance Tips."

Then, in a controlled motion, slowly lower your forearms back to the floor. Feel some of the tension release from your lower back, and repeat.

PERFORMANCE TIPS

- Start with four repetitions, holding each for 4 seconds. The next week, do five reps of 4 seconds each.

- If you have a strong lower back, you may need to hold for longer than the number of seconds recommended here to feel the exercise do its work.

- Keep your torso and neck in the same position throughout the exercise.

- Don't hold your breath. Breathe normally. You can even count the seconds of each contraction with your breathing, taking one strong breath per second.

GET THE RESULTS YOU WANT

The last time you watched the Summer Olympics, chances are, the sprinters had the muscles you most admired.

Now think about what a sprinter does to get those muscles. He runs really fast for short distances (duh); and he lifts weights . . . just like you do. Both of those are anaerobic exercises. *Anaerobic* means that your body can't use oxygen to release the fuel it needs for energy, because the exercises don't make your heart and lungs work hard enough to quickly move the oxygen. So you have to use other energy systems. One alternative system uses a substance in your muscles called creatine phosphate. It lasts just 30 seconds or less. The second uses glycogen, a sugar stored in your muscles. It can provide energy for up to 3 minutes in the most highly conditioned athletes, although for most people 60 to 100 seconds is probably the limit.

Weight lifting is like sprinting in both intensity and duration, and thus uses the anaerobic energy systems, relying very little on the aerobic energy system. Thus, if you add a sprint workout to your three weekly weight workouts in Level Three of the Core Program, you get four anaerobic training sessions a week.

Why is that good? Well, let's go back to the example of the Olympic athletes. Which physiques did you admire least? I'd bet you didn't want to look like the marathoners, who do aerobic workouts. You wouldn't be reading a book about building arm muscles if you wanted to look like you'd just been released from a gulag.

So you want to look more like the sprinters, who do anaerobic workouts, and less like the marathoners, who do aerobic workouts. That brings up a tricky issue. Aerobic exercise provides astounding benefits for health and longevity. And so far, strength-training research has failed to show that anaerobic exercise helps you live longer.

The solution is to continue doing two aerobic workouts each week while adding a sprint workout that bridges the gap between aerobic and anaerobic. You do anaerobic work during the sprints, but move continuously in between sprints, getting a mild aerobic workout too.

This is an advanced plan. Beginners should stay on the same path as in Levels One and Two, working up to 20 continuous minutes in their target heart-rate zone.

The Beginner Plan

Here's a 32-minute program for Week 1 of Level Three.

- 5 minutes at easy pace
- 10 minutes at target pace
- 2 minutes at easy pace
- 10 minutes at target pace
- 5 minutes at easy pace

For Week 2, do a half-hour workout with 20 consecutive minutes at your target heart rate.

- 5 minutes at easy pace
- 20 minutes at target pace
- 5 minutes at easy pace

■ If I do two sets of each arm and leg exercise except the forearm exercises, that's a total of 20 sets per workout. Who has that kind of time?
You can shorten the workout and still get the desired effects by doing supersets of the arm exercises. Supersets are simply sets done at full intensity but without any rest between them.

Warm up using about one-half to two-thirds of the weight you'd normally use on each exercise. Do the three triceps exercises consecutively, and then without resting, immediately follow them with the three biceps exercises.

Then let it rip—do one full-intensity superset for triceps and one for biceps. Follow that with a forearm superset. You don't need a warmup for your forearms; just go all-out on your one superset. This will make your workout about 13 minutes shorter than if you took 60-second rests.

Finally, do your leg exercises the normal way—two sets of each, resting for 30 to 60 seconds in between sets and exercises.

■ I've made big jumps in the amount of weight I use on all these exercises. But I don't see bigger muscles in the mirror. Why not?
If you're lifting weights for the first time or following a long layoff, your body is doing exactly what it's supposed to do. As explained in the troubleshooting feature in Level Two, the first adjustment your body makes is to recruit more muscle fibers and nerve cells. This is called neuromuscular learning, and it makes you stronger but not necessarily bigger.

Rest assured, the next step is bigger muscles. The great thing about the strength you're adding now is that it enables you to handle bigger weights, and that means more muscle down the road.

■ I've really enjoyed this program, except now it's the 6th week and I'm really sick of doing those same overhead triceps extensions and biceps curls that I started doing in Level One.
This is why no workout routine should last longer than 6 to 8 weeks without changes. By the end of the 6th week, your body has probably made all the adjustments it's going to make via the exercises you started doing in Level One—especially if you came to the Core Program with some recent weight-lifting experience. And, obviously, your mind is ready for a change.

So now it's time to turn the page, both figuratively and literally. Chapter 12 will show you some keys to a lifetime of success in weight training, and chapter 13 will show you advanced arm-building workouts. You should find plenty of new exercises and routines there. Your muscles will appreciate the new challenges, and your brain will enjoy having something new to get it pumped up.

The Advanced Plan

For your first cardio workout each week, do the following sprint routine. Running is ideal, although you can also do sprints on a bike or in a swimming pool. Or use a jump rope for your sprints and jog in place in between them. Once you've picked your exercise, do this:

- 5 minutes at easy pace (Take a brisk walk or light jog if you're running)
- 10 seconds at hard pace—go as fast as you can
- 2 minutes at easy pace (Walk or jog, if you're a runner)
- Repeat for a total of 10 sprints and recovery periods
- 5 minutes at easy pace for a cooldown, doing whatever you did to warm up (The 2 minutes at easy pace after your final sprint can count as part of this cooldown)

For your second heart-healthy workout of the week, do a traditional aerobic workout.

- 5 minutes at easy pace
- 20 minutes at target rate
- 5 minutes at easy pace

For your third aerobic workout, do the interval workout introduced in Level Two.

- 5 minutes at easy pace
- 30 seconds at hard pace—not all-out like a sprint but the best effort you can put out for 30 seconds
- 1 minute at easy pace (Just take a brisk walk or light jog if you're running, or drop a couple of levels on a cardio machine)
- Repeat for a total of 8 to 12 intervals and recovery periods
- 5 minutes at easy pace for a cooldown (The 1-minute at easy pace during your final interval can count as part of this cooldown)

EATING ESSENTIALS:
A COMPLETE MUSCLE-BUILDING DIET

It's time to integrate all the components of your diet—fat and carbohydrates as well as protein—to ensure the best mix for health, energy, and longevity.

Protein

As discussed in chapter 9, guys who lift weights should shoot for an intake of 7 to 10 grams of protein for every 10 pounds of body weight. If you err with your protein intake, it should be on the high side. There isn't any danger in eating a little more than your body can use to build muscle during periods of intense exercise (if, indeed, this amount really is more than your body can use—a question that's open to debate).

What happens to the excess? Your body eliminates it or possibly uses some of it for fuel during exercise. Either way, your body uses a lot of energy to process it, and that alone speeds up your metabolism.

Fat

Decades of good science have shown that cutting fat out of your diet will help you lose weight. Fat has 9 calories per gram, which means it packs more than twice as many calories in the same space as either protein or carbohydrates does.

And yet, people who go on high-fat, low-carbohydrate diets almost always lose weight. These diets were used to great effect by bodybuilders in the pre-steroid era. These old-timers weren't quick-fix guys—they simply knew that a diet consisting almost entirely of fat and protein allowed them to build muscle while shedding fat.

Giving ammunition to the pro-fat gurus is research showing tremendous health benefits from certain kinds of fat. Monounsaturated fat, for example, can lower LDL cholesterol (the bad kind) while raising HDL (the good kind). This is the type of fat found in olives and olive oil, nuts, seeds, and avocados. Polyunsaturated fat, such as that found in fish and fish oils, can also improve cholesterol and thus lower your risk of heart disease.

No health benefits have been associated with the other types of fat: saturated (found in animal products like meat, dairy foods, and eggs and in coconut, palm, and palm kernel oils) and hydrogenated or trans fats (found in margarine, mayonnaise, and most prepared bakery products like doughnuts, pie crusts, and muffins). These fats are the hardest for your body to digest and use for energy, and are most associated with obesity and heart disease.

I recommend that you make fat 30 to 40 percent of your total diet. But most of that should be monounsaturated and polyunsaturated fats. Add fats like olive oil to your diet: Use full-fat oil-based salad dressings, for example. Minimize saturated fats by eating low-fat dairy products and the leanest meats you can find. And try to do

without hydrogenated fats altogether—sorry, but you should stop eating doughnuts and pies except as very occasional treats.

Carbohydrates

The big, bad problem associated with carbohydrates is that they cause your body to release more insulin. Extra insulin is great after exercise, when you need it to speed nutrients to your muscles for refueling and repair. But it's bad when the insulin doesn't have anything to do but cause your body to store fat. Insulin also makes you hungrier faster, which is the drawback of low-fat, high-carbohydrate diets.

If you ate a 40-percent-protein, 40-percent-fat diet, carbohydrates would make up the remaining 20 percent. You'd probably lose a lot of weight on this diet, if for no other reason than that the protein and fat would make you feel full most of the time.

On the other hand, if you ate a 20-percent-protein, 30-percent-fat diet, you'd eat 50 percent carbohydrates. This is a good diet for gaining muscular weight. The carbohydrates give you plenty of readily available energy for workouts and also help you maintain a healthy appetite—a must if you're trying to pack on solid weight.

The best carbohydrates come from fruits (try berries, citrus fruits, and kiwifruit), vegetables (go for a mix of colors, such as red tomatoes, orange carrots, and green peas), beans (they have lots of fiber, which makes you feel full and thus is vital to a weight-loss diet), and whole-grain breads and pasta (the right kind has "whole wheat flour" as the first ingredient on the label, as opposed to the kind that leads off with "enriched flour").

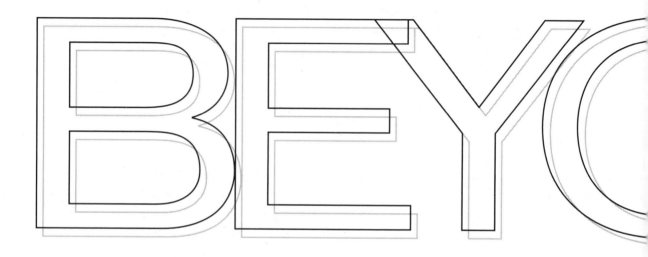

PART FOUR

OND
THE CORE
PROGRAM

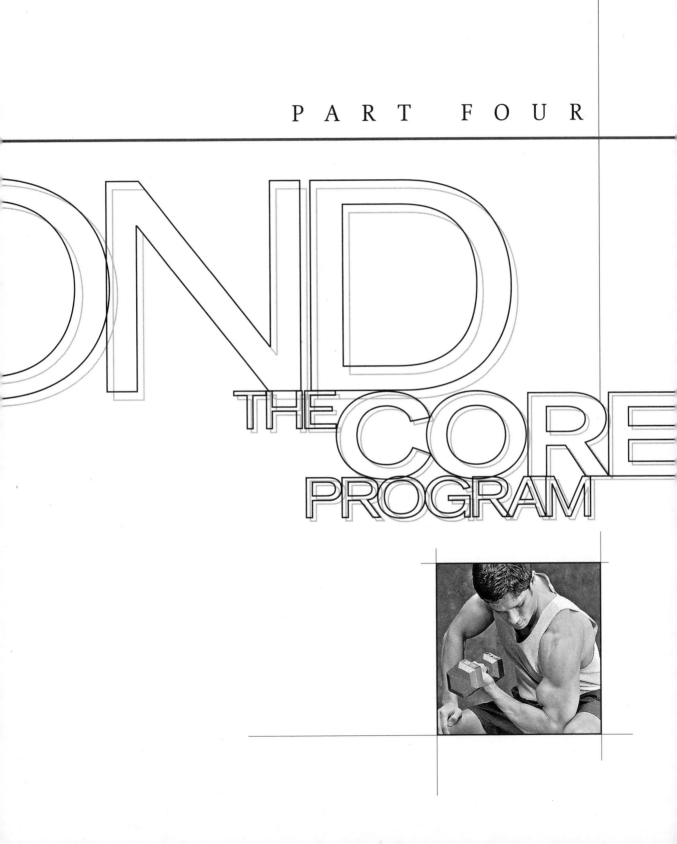

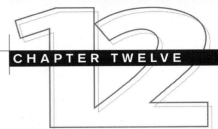

CHAPTER TWELVE

ESSENTIAL MAINTENANCE

Your arms look and feel quite a bit different than they did 6 weeks ago—bigger, stronger, more defined. When you flex, your biceps pop; when you straighten your arm again, your triceps undulate. Go stand in front of a mirror and try it, if you don't believe me.

And those are just the improvements in your arms—your entire body should feel tighter and more powerful. If you were heavy to begin with, you've probably dropped a few pounds, especially from your waist. You eat better during the day and sleep better at night.

So what the hell do you do next? Here are a few ideas about how to hold on to or even build on the gains that you've made in the past 6 weeks.

ARM EXERCISE

Still interested in making your arm muscles bigger? You don't need to do any more exercises than you did in Level Three. You just need to make these movements increasingly tougher on your arm muscles. Here are a few ways to accomplish that.

■ Play the angles. Any exercise that you can do sitting or standing straight up, you can do leaning forward or back. A simple biceps curl becomes a different and more difficult exercise when you lean your torso back on an inclined exercise bench. Or you can flip around, lay your chest on the incline bench, and do the exercise leaning forward.

- Change up your triceps exercises too. Rather than sit straight up while doing overhead triceps extensions, you can lean back on an incline bench. Or you can lie on your back on a flat bench. In that case, you wouldn't lower the weights behind your head but would instead start with your arms perpendicular to your torso, straight up over your shoulders. Another option is to lie on a decline bench.
- Experiment. See what other guys in the gym are doing, and see what works for you. As explained in chapter 6, change is the one constant you need in your workouts to keep getting better results.
- Get stronger. Many guys see the biggest increases in arm size when they focus on strength-building exercises like bench presses and bent-over rows. Although your arms are only helper muscles in these exercises, which focus on your chest and back, they get a tremendous growth stimulus from the heavy weights you use.

So, a couple of times a year, focus on pure strength. That is, try to improve your maximum bench press, and make sure you do the same number of sets and rows for your back muscles, at the same intensity. In other words, when you do max-

imum-weight bench presses, make sure you do maximum-weight bent-over rows too.

Whatever variations you choose, remember that muscle growth is a moving target. The more experienced you are, the faster your body adapts to what you're doing. Never continue with any program longer than six workouts without making some sort of change.

AEROBICS

If your only goal is building muscle, you don't want to exceed the amount of aerobic exercise you did in the Core Program, whether you did the beginner workouts or the advanced techniques.

But if you want to improve your aerobic fitness—and burn off a few more calories—you can increase to five aerobic workouts a week. One of these should be a completely different activity from your usual routine. If you usually jog, swim laps instead; if you're a cyclist, go for a power walk; if you play handball, try one of those stairclimbing machines. The point is to rest the muscles you usually use, recruit some new muscles for a change, and—perhaps most important—prevent boredom from setting in.

If you still have some weight to lose while you're trying to gain muscle, try the advanced interval and sprint workouts described, respectively, in Levels Two and Three of the Core Program, if you haven't already.

Another technique for accelerating fat

loss with aerobic exercise is called multi-mode training. This works if you belong to a gym and don't prefer any one form of cardio exercise over another. Try a 5-minute warmup on one machine—a treadmill, say—and then go harder for 5 to 10 minutes. Then stop the treadmill, step off, and do a completely different machine—a rowing machine, for example—for the next 10 minutes. Finish with 10 minutes on a third machine, such as an elliptical machine or stationary bike, and then cool down for 5 minutes on that same machine.

Using different machines in the same workout forces your body to make continual adjustments. You never hit a comfortable groove. That makes the exercise harder and thus more beneficial than a steady workout on one machine.

EATING

The Core Program laid out a diet plan that you can follow for life to stay lean and energetic. Here are a few more suggestions about managing your diet to get the body you want.

Manage your weight with the 15/500 rule. If despite your 6 weeks of exercise you could still stand to lose a few pounds, cut your daily food intake by no more than 15 percent or 500 calories, whichever is the lesser amount. Restricting calories by any more will slow down your metabolism, actually preventing weight loss.

If you're still a relatively scrawny guy who wants to bulk up, increase your daily feed by the lesser of 15 percent or 500 calories.

Pack a snack. As evidenced by your need for pre- and postworkout snacks, hoisting dumbbells makes you hungry. You'll probably need food every 2 to 3 hours throughout the day. That's healthful *food*, not an entire meal or a bar of sugar from a vending machine or a paper carton of fried grease from a drive-thru. Grab some fruits, nuts, or even peanut butter and jelly on whole grain bread. And keep a stash in your briefcase, desk, or gym bag for emergency munching.

Don't go to sleep on an empty stomach. If you have dinner at 6:00 P.M. and have a snack 3 hours later, at 9:00, you're still due for another feeding before bedtime. This one is especially important because it will prevent your body from cannibalizing your hard-won muscle tissue while you're unconscious. Keep your bedtime snack to about 500 calories, and make sure it's not too heavy on the protein. A beef-and-bean burrito right before bed will give you not only gas but also intense dreams that will wake you up just in time to smell it.

CHAPTER THIRTEEN

ESSENTIAL ADVANCED ROUTINES

The eight biceps and triceps arm-pumping exercises you learned in the Core Program are just a small sampling of the possibilities. Here are six new routines you can enlist to keep augmenting your arms.

1. A four-exercise dumbbell routine that offers advanced versions of the exercises you learned in the Core Program
2. A six-exercise using a cable-crossover machine
3. A four-exercise barbell routine
4. A three-exercise routine to improve your performance when you play sports
5. A six-exercise superset routine
6. A two-exercise body-weight routine you can do at home, in a gym, or on a playground

Each routine also includes a training log in which you can track the sets and reps you do each workout.

MASTER CLASS

If you liked the exercises in the Core Program, here's how you can continue doing them and still see benefits. These are advanced versions of four exercises you just finished doing. Do this routine twice a week, using a 4-week cycle.

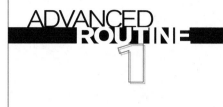

Week 1: Do one set of 12 to 15 repetitions of each exercise.

Week 2: Do two sets of 8 to 12 repetitions of each.

Week 3: Do three sets of 4 to 8 repetitions of each.

Week 4: Do three sets of each exercise, with 12 to 15 reps in set one, 8 to 12 in set two, and 4 to 8 in set three.

MASTER-CLASS TRAINING LOG

Master-Class Exercises	WEEK 1		WEEK 2		WEEK 3		WEEK 4	
	Workout 1	Workout 2	Workout 1	Workout 2	Workout 1	Workout 2	Workout 1	Workout 2
One-arm dumbbell extension								
Kickback with rotation								
Incline dumbbell curl								
Concentration curl								

One-Arm Dumbbell Extension

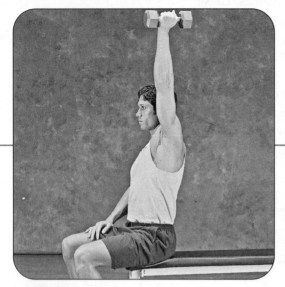

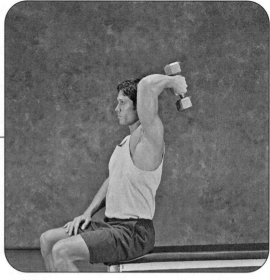

READY, SET:

Sit on a weight bench and, with your nondominant hand, hold a dumbbell straight overhead. Your palm should face in toward you, and your upper arm should be next to your ear.

GO:

Slowly bend your elbow to lower the weight behind you as far as you can without moving your upper arm.

Pause, then slowly lift the weight back to the starting position. Repeat. When you finish all of your repetitions with your nondominant arm, hold the weight in your dominant hand and do the same number of reps with that arm.

PERFORMANCE TIPS

■ This exercise can be a little tough on your elbows, especially the first few times, since you won't be used to working one arm at a time in an overhead exercise. Make sure you work slowly—never lower the weight quickly and jerk it back up.

■ The key, as with all overhead triceps exercises, is to keep your upper arm stationary, as close to perpendicular to the floor as you can. You can support your upper arm with your free hand, if you want.

Kickback with Rotation

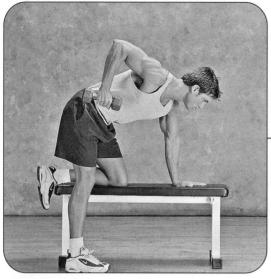

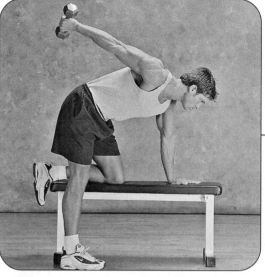

READY, SET:

Hold a dumbbell with your nondominant hand, palm facing in. Put your opposite hand and knee on the bench so that your body is at about a 90-degree angle. Your back should be flat and parallel to the bench and the floor. Raise the dumbbell straight up to the side of your abdomen, and point your elbow up toward the ceiling.

GO:

Keeping your elbow pointing straight up, slowly straighten your arm, lifting the weight as high as you can toward the ceiling while rotating your wrist upward (pronating) so your palm faces upward at the end of the movement. Pause to feel the squeeze in your triceps.

Slowly lower the weight back to the starting position, rotating your wrist back inward (supinating), and repeat. When you finish all of your repetitions with your nondominant arm, hold the weight in your dominant hand and do the same number of reps with that arm.

PERFORMANCE TIPS

■ Start with your weaker arm, and do the same number of reps on each side.

■ Keep your elbow pointed up toward the ceiling throughout the exercise.

Incline Dumbbell Curl

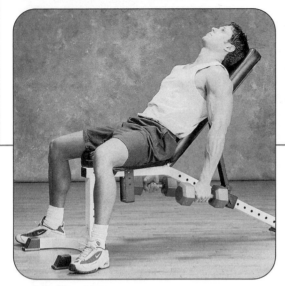 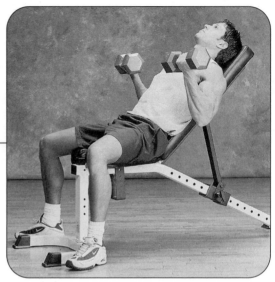

READY, SET:

Set an incline bench to an angle between 45 and 70 degrees to the floor. Hold a pair of dumbbells, sit on the bench with your back resting against the pad, and let your arms hang straight down from your shoulders.

GO:

Without moving your upper arms, bend your elbows to lift the weights toward your shoulders. As the weights move past your thighs, rotate your wrists upward (supinate) so your palms face your shoulders at the end of the movement. Stop when you've lifted the weights as high as you can without moving your upper arms.

Pause, then slowly lower the weights back to the starting position, rotating your wrists downward (pronating) until they're in the original position. Repeat.

PERFORMANCE TIPS

■ Your head position is a matter of comfort. Some guys rest their heads against the pad, others keep them upright.

■ The lower the incline, the tougher this exercise will be on your shoulders. So if you feel discomfort in your shoulder sockets, try raising the bench a bit.

Concentration Curl

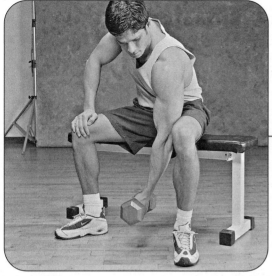 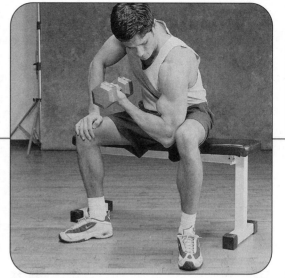

READY, SET:

Sit on the bench with your knees spread wide, and hold a dumbbell with your nondominant hand. Bend forward and rest that elbow against your inner thigh, down by your knee. Rest your free hand on your other knee. Lower the weight until your arm hangs straight down from your shoulder, with your palm out.

GO:

Without moving your upper arm, slowly bend your elbow to lift the weight as high as you can. Pause to feel the squeeze in your biceps.

Slowly lower the weight back to the starting position, rotating your wrist back inward (pronating), and repeat. When you finish all of your repetitions with your nondominant arm, hold the weight in your dominant hand and do the same number of reps with that arm.

PERFORMANCE TIPS

■ Keep your body in one position throughout the exercise; your lower arm should be your only moving part. As you start using heavier weights, you'll be tempted to lean back to finish some of the repetitions, but that just takes work away from your biceps.

CROSSOVER POTENTIAL

The cable-crossover machine is one of the most versatile contraptions in the gym. With both high and low
cables and two separate weight stacks, you can work any
muscle in your body, and the only limit to the exercises'
effectiveness is your imagination.

Do the following routine once or twice a week, using
this 4-week cycle.

Week 1: Do one set of 12 to 15 repetitions of each exercise.

Week 2: Do two sets of 8 to 12 repetitions of each.

Week 3: Do three sets of 4 to 8 repetitions of each.

Week 4: Do three sets of each exercise, with 12 to 15
reps in set one, 8 to 12 reps in set two, and 4 to 8 reps in
set three.

ADVANCED
ROUTINE
2

CROSSOVER-POTENTIAL TRAINING LOG

Crossover-Potential Exercises	WEEK 1		WEEK 2		WEEK 3		WEEK 4	
	Workout 1	Workout 2	Workout 1	Workout 2	Workout 1	Workout 2	Workout 1	Workout 2
Double cross pulldown								
High-cable kickback								
High-cable double curl								
High-cable overhead triceps extension								
Low-cable reverse curl								
Low-cable double curl								

Double Cross Pulldown

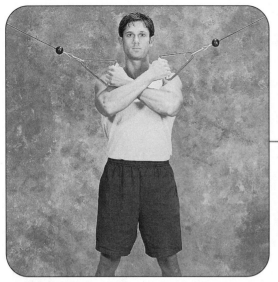

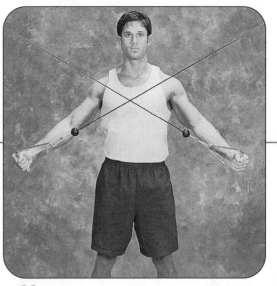

READY, SET:

Attach stirrup handles to the high cable pulleys. Grab the left handle with your right hand and the right handle with your left hand. Stand in the middle of the crossover station in an athletic posture—feet shoulder-width apart, knees slightly bent. Hold the handles up near your chin (right hand near left side of chin, left near right), with your palms facing your body and your elbows bent.

GO:

Without moving your upper arms, slowly pull the handles down and away from your body. Pause to feel the squeeze in your triceps.

Slowly bend your elbows to return back to the starting position, and repeat.

PERFORMANCE TIPS

■ Keep your upper arms in one position throughout the exercise.
If you move them up and down, you use muscles in your back and shoulders in the exercise.

■ Also keep your shoulders in one position throughout the exercise.
If you allow them to shrug up and down, you take work away from your triceps.

High-Cable Kickback

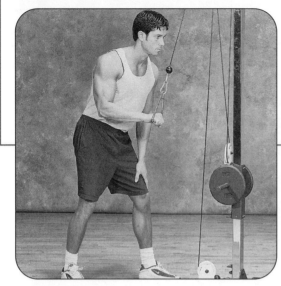 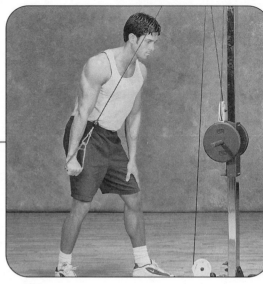

READY, SET:

Turn your body toward one of the weight stacks. Using an overhand grip, grab one of the high-pulley stirrup handles with your nondominant hand. Bend forward at the waist, and brace your free hand on your corresponding knee. Bend your working elbow 90 degrees, and keep your upper arm pressed against your side.

GO:

Without moving your upper arm, slowly pull the handle down and back. Pause to feel the squeeze in your triceps.

Slowly bend your elbow to return back to the starting position, and repeat. When you finish all of your repetitions with your nondominant arm, hold the handle in your dominant hand and do the same number of reps with that arm.

PERFORMANCE TIPS

■ Keep your body in one position throughout the exercise; your elbow should be your only moving part.

■ Start with your weaker arm—probably your left, if you're right-handed.

High-Cable Double Curl

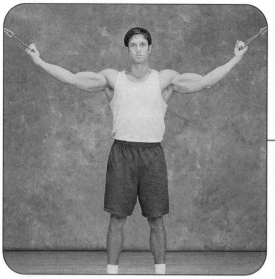
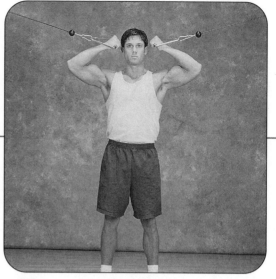

READY, SET:

Attach stirrup handles to the high cable pulleys. Using an underhand grip, grab the right handle with your right hand and the left handle with your left. Stand in the middle of the crossover station in an athletic posture—feet shoulder-width apart, knees slightly bent. Hold your upper arms parallel to the floor, with your palms facing up.

GO:

Without moving your upper arms, slowly bend your elbows to pull the handles toward your ears. Pause to feel the squeeze in your biceps.

Slowly straighten your arms to return back to the starting position, and repeat.

PERFORMANCE TIPS

- Keep your upper arms stationary throughout the exercise; your elbows should be your only moving parts.

- For an interesting variation, try bringing your hands behind your head on each repetition. You'll have to start with your arms at a different angle—your elbows will point up a bit, rather than straight out to the sides.

- If you find that you're moving your body too much while standing to do this exercise, you can try it while sitting on a weight bench or even kneeling on the floor.

High-Cable Overhead Triceps Extension

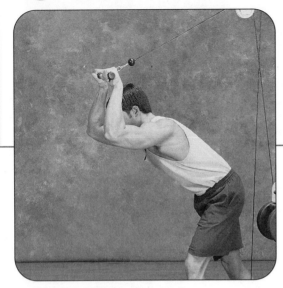 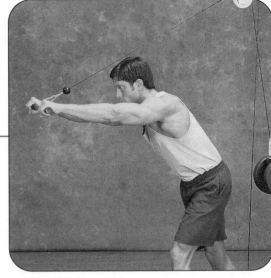

READY, SET:

Attach a straight bar to a high cable pulley. Grab the bar with an overhand grip, with your hands about 12 inches apart. Turn your back to the weight stack and stand with one foot in front of the other (it doesn't matter which one is forward). Bend forward at the waist so your back is at a 45-degree angle to the floor. Hold the bar above your head, with your elbows bent 90 degrees and pointed forward.

GO:

Slowly straighten your arms. Pause to feel the squeeze in your triceps.

Slowly bend your elbows to return back to the starting position, and repeat.

PERFORMANCE TIPS

■ As with any single-joint triceps exercise, keep your body in one position throughout the exercise; your elbows should be your only moving parts.

■ Most guys allow their upper arms to move backward when returning to the starting position at the end of a repetition, then move them forward again at the start of the next rep. This is an easy way to generate extra momentum, but it transfers work from your triceps to your lats.

Low-Cable Reverse Curl

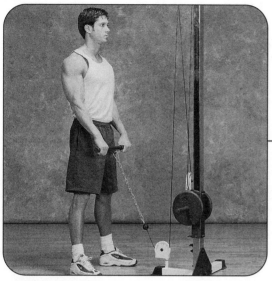

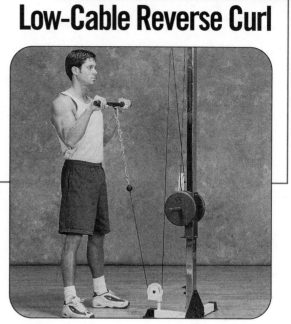

READY, SET:

Attach a straight bar to a low cable pulley. Grab the bar with an overhand grip and stand facing the weight stack, about 1½ feet away from it. Hold the bar in front of your thighs, at arm's length, with your upper arms pressed against your sides, your shoulders back, your feet shoulder-width apart, and your knees slightly bent.

GO:

Slowly bend your elbows to pull the bar toward your chest.

Pause, then slowly straighten your arms to return to the starting position. Repeat.

PERFORMANCE TIPS

■ Keep your upper arms pressed against your sides throughout the movement. If you let them drift out to the sides, your shoulders end up lifting the weight.

■ Likewise, keep your knees slightly bent and your back in its natural alignment throughout the exercise. If you unbalance your body with locked knees or an overly straightened or curved back, you'll probably rock back and forth, using your whole body to generate momentum and taking work away from your biceps and forearms.

Low-Cable Double Curl

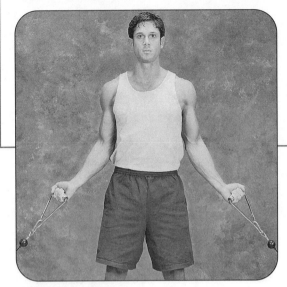

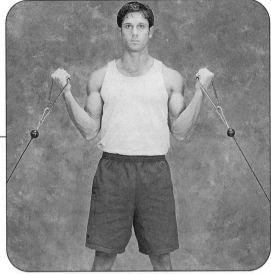

READY, SET:

Attach stirrup handles to the low cable pulleys. Using an underhand grip, grab the right handle with your right hand and the left handle with your left. Stand in the middle of the crossover station in an athletic posture—feet shoulder-width apart, knees slightly bent. Press your upper arms against your sides.

GO:

Slowly bend your elbows to pull the handles toward your shoulders.

Pause, then slowly straighten your arms to return to the starting position. Repeat.

PERFORMANCE TIPS

■ Keep your upper arms pressed against your sides throughout the exercise. If you let them drift out to the sides, your shoulders end up lifting the weights.

■ You can create any number of slight variations on this exercise by standing farther forward or back relative to the crossover station. You can also change the angle by sitting on a weight bench or even kneeling on the floor.

THE BARBELL ROUTINE

The biceps and triceps are among the simplest muscles in your body, in both form and function. So they're a perfect match for the simplest bodybuilding tool: the barbell. The following four-exercise routine gives your arm muscles some serious work. All you need are a barbell, a bench, and a room where you're free to sweat, grunt, and occasionally use language you wouldn't want your children to repeat.

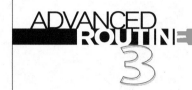

Do this routine twice a week for a 4-week cycle.

Week 1: Do one set of 12 to 15 repetitions of each exercise.

Week 2: Do two sets of 8 to 12 repetitions of each.

Week 3: Do three sets of 4 to 8 repetitions of each.

Week 4: Do three sets of each exercise, with 12 to 15 reps in set one, 8 to 12 reps in set two, and 4 to 8 reps in set three.

BARBELL-ROUTINE TRAINING LOG

Barbell-Routine Exercises	WEEK 1		WEEK 2		WEEK 3		WEEK 4	
	Workout 1	Workout 2	Workout 1	Workout 2	Workout 1	Workout 2	Workout 1	Workout 2
Lying barbell extension								
Close-grip bench press								
Barbell curl								
Barbell concentration curl								

Lying Barbell Extension

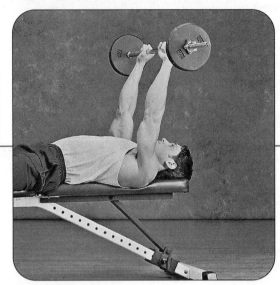

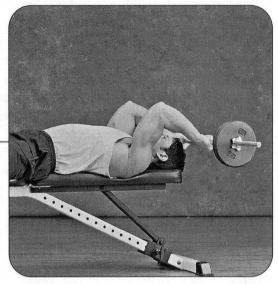

READY, SET:

Grab the barbell with an overhand, shoulder-width grip. Lie on the weight bench with your feet flat on the floor for stability. Hold the bar straight over your forehead. Tuck your chin toward your chest so your weight rests on your shoulder blades.

GO:

Without moving your upper arms, slowly lower the bar behind you until your elbows are bent 90 degrees.

Pause, then slowly lift the bar back to the starting position. Repeat.

PERFORMANCE TIPS

■ Keep your upper arms in one position throughout the exercise.

■ This exercise is often called a skull crusher in gyms; indeed, one variation of the exercise is to start with the bar over your chest and lower it to your forehead. Although that's a great drill for teaching you to lower the bar slowly and under control (failure to do so explains the nickname), it's a tough angle on your elbows. It's far better to start with your upper arms angled back slightly, as shown here.

Close-Grip Bench Press

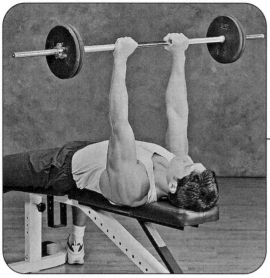

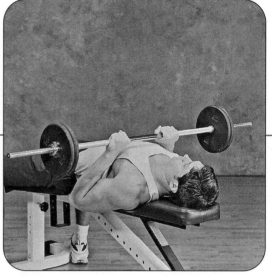

READY, SET:

Grab the bar with an overhand grip, with your hands 6 to 12 inches apart (the closer position can be uncomfortable for your wrists). Lie on the bench with your feet flat on the floor for stability. Hold the bar straight above your chest.

GO:

Slowly lower the bar to the bottom of your chest (or within an inch of it).

Pause, then slowly lift the bar back to the starting position. Repeat.

PERFORMANCE TIPS

■ Keep your body stable throughout the exercise; don't arch your back to push the weight off your chest.

■ This is one of the few multijoint triceps exercises. (The bench dip is another.) Your upper arms are supposed to move, so the shoulder joints are engaged along with the elbow joints. The advantage to multijoint exercises is that you can use more weight and thus give your triceps a more intense muscle-building stimulus. When you do low-repetition sets with heavy weights, make sure you use a spotter who can pull the bar off your chest if you run out of gas.

■ Many guys do supersets of lying barbell extensions and close-grip bench presses, without changing weights. When the triceps are fatigued from the extensions, they go immediately into close-grip benches without stopping. That produces a deeper level of fatigue in the triceps than results from normal sets of these exercises.

Barbell Curl

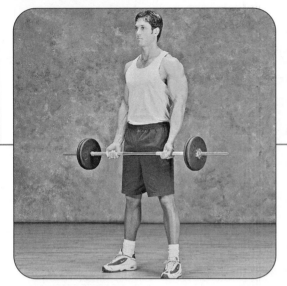 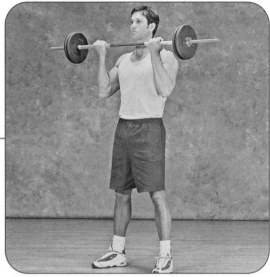

READY, SET:

Grab the barbell with an underhand grip, with your hands just wider than shoulder-width apart. Hold the bar in front of your thighs, at arm's length, with your upper arms pressed against your sides, your shoulders back, your feet shoulder-width apart, and your knees slightly bent.

GO:

Without moving your upper arms, slowly bend your elbows to lift the bar toward your chin. At the top of the movement, when your forearms are perpendicular to the floor, elevate your elbows slightly and feel the squeeze in your biceps.

Slowly lower the bar back to the starting position, and repeat.

PERFORMANCE TIPS

■ This is one of the most notorious "cheat" exercises in the gym; you always see guys leaning forward and back to generate momentum that allows them to use weights heavier than their biceps can handle. Stick to a weight you can lift smoothly, with your torso stationary and your knees unlocked.

■ The wider your grip on the bar, the more you'll work the inner—or short—head of the biceps. And the closer your grip, the more you'll work the inner—or long—head, along with the brachialis. So if you do three sets, you can change the width of your grip for each set.

Barbell Concentration Curl

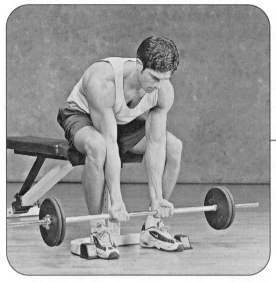 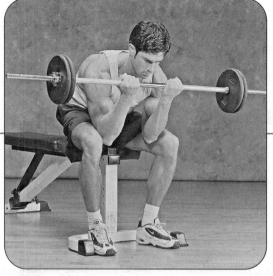

READY, SET:

Grab the barbell with a narrow, underhand grip, with your hands 4 to 6 inches apart. Sit on the end of the bench with your feet about 12 inches apart, and lean forward until your upper body is nearly parallel to the floor. Your elbows should touch the insides of your knees but not rest on them. Let your arms hang straight down toward the floor.

GO:

Without moving your upper arms, slowly bend your elbows to lift the bar toward your chin.

Pause, then slowly lower the bar back to the starting position. Repeat.

PERFORMANCE TIPS

- The concentration curl is aptly named; when you do it right, you focus fully on how your biceps feel throughout each repetition.

- Keep your elbows in contact with your knees throughout the exercise.

- Keep your head in line with your torso and your eyes looking down toward the floor. Maintain this head and torso position throughout the exercise.

THE SPORTS ROUTINE

Big ol' muscles are great for impressing women, intimidating men, and juggling small children. But they won't help you much in sports unless they're combined with balance, coordination, and endurance.

The following three moves will help you in each of those areas. The farmer's carry improves forearm endurance, while the triangle pushup on a ball and the kung fu curl on one leg develop balance and coordination. And, fair warning, all three will draw some pretty odd stares from passersby if you do them in a gym.

Do this routine once or twice a week for a month.

SPORTS-ROUTINE TRAINING LOG

Sports-Routine Exercises	WEEK 1		WEEK 2		WEEK 3		WEEK 4	
	Workout 1	Workout 2	Workout 1	Workout 2	Workout 1	Workout 2	Workout 1	Workout 2
Farmer's carry								
Pushup on ball								
Kung fu curl on one leg								

Farmer's Carry

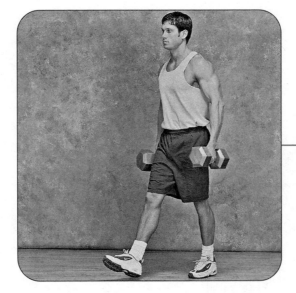

READY, SET, GO:

Grab a pair of dumbbells that, together, add up to half of your body weight. (If you weigh 180 pounds, start with two 45-pound dumbbells.) Hold them at your sides. Walk for 20 seconds in one direction, stop, set the weights down, rest for 5 seconds, then pick them up and walk back to the starting point. That's one rep.

PERFORMANCE TIPS

■ Do three sets as described above, walking for 20 seconds in each direction.

■ When you can do this exercise while holding dumbbells that total your body weight, try it while walking on tiptoe.

■ A challenging variation is to carry, in each hand, a weight plate—preferably a bumper plate, which has a lip you can use for a handhold.

Pushup on Ball

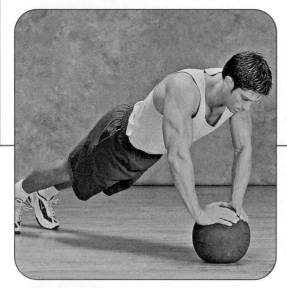

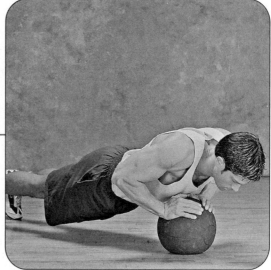

READY, SET:

Grab a basketball or medicine ball and set it on the floor. Get into a pushup position with your hands on the ball. Your forefingers and thumbs should touch or nearly touch, forming a diamond shape. Position your body in a straight line from your neck to your heels. Straighten your arms over the ball.

GO:

Bend your elbows to lower your body toward the ball. When your chest touches or nearly touches it, pause.

Then push back up to return to the starting position, and repeat.

PERFORMANCE TIPS

- Do three sets of 8 to 12 repetitions.

- This is a very tough exercise to master. If you can't do more than a few repetitions, finish your set by doing pushups on the floor, with your hands in the same diamond shape. If those are too easy, elevate your feet on a bench.

Kung Fu Curl on One Leg

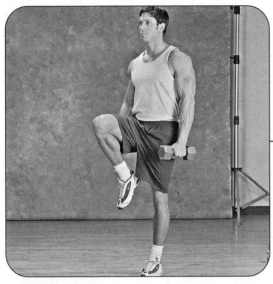

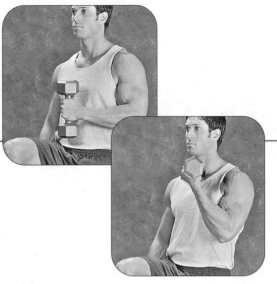

READY, SET:

Grab a pair of dumbbells and hold them with your arms hanging straight down from your shoulders. Lift your right leg until your thigh is parallel to the floor, with your knee bent.

GO:

Lift the weight in your left hand toward your belly button.

KEEP GOING . . .

Continue lifting the weight to your shoulder, rotating your wrist inward (supinating).

Lower the weight back to your abs, rotating your wrist back outward (pronating). Then continue lowering back to the starting position, and repeat. When you finish all of your repetitions with your left arm, switch position: Lower your right leg, raise your left leg, and do the same number of reps with your right arm.

PERFORMANCE TIPS

- Do three sets of 8 to 12 repetitions.

- You may want to try a two-feet-on-the-floor version of the exercise first. Curl the weights alternately, lifting the weight in your right hand as soon as you've lowered the weight in your left. Aim for a smooth, synchronous movement.

THE SUPERSET ROUTINE

Instead of resting after every set of every exercise, put together multiple sets of different exercises before resting. Do a set of a biceps exercise followed immediately by a set of a triceps exercise, without rest in between. Then rest for 30 to 60 seconds and either repeat the superset or move on to the next one. Besides saving time, supersets induce deeper exhaustion in your muscles.

Try these three pairs of exercises on a 4-week cycle.

Week 1: Do one superset of each exercise pair, with 12 to 15 repetitions per set of each exercise.

Week 2: Do two supersets, with 8 to 12 repetitions per set of each exercise.

Week 3: Do three supersets, with 4 to 8 repetitions per set of each exercise.

Week 4: Do three supersets, one with 12 to 15 reps per set of each exercise, a second with 8 to 12 reps per set of each exercise, and a third with 4 to 8 reps per set of each exercise.

SUPERSET-ROUTINE TRAINING LOG

Superset-Routine Exercises	WEEK 1		WEEK 2		WEEK 3		WEEK 4	
	Workout 1	Workout 2	Workout 1	Workout 2	Workout 1	Workout 2	Workout 1	Workout 2
Preacher curl								
Decline triceps extension								
Reverse curl								
Cable pushdown								
Standing high-cable curl								
Cable reverse pushdown								

Preacher Curl

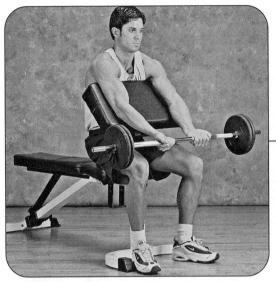 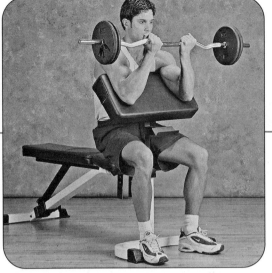

READY, SET:

Grab an EZ-curl bar with a medium-width, under-hand grip and position yourself in the preacher-curl station so the top of the pad reaches your armpits when you sit on the bench. Lay your upper arms flat on the pad and extend your arms.

GO:

Slowly bend your elbows to lift the bar until your elbows are at about a 90-degree angle.

Pause, then slowly lower the bar back to the starting position. Repeat.

PERFORMANCE TIPS

- Keep constant tension on your biceps. After you lift the weight to a certain point—usually if you bend your elbows to an angle that's smaller than 90 degrees—you aren't working against gravity anymore, and your muscles don't have to work much to hold the weight. Stop the exercise before you reach that point.

- This is a favorite exercise of the bodybuilders in the gym, who put their upper bodies through all sorts of contortions to lift heavier weights. Ignore the impulse to pile on the plates; use only as much weight as you can handle with perfect form for the recommended number of repetitions.

Decline Triceps Extension

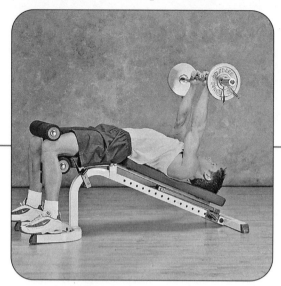 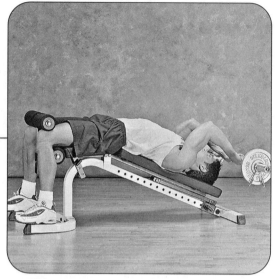

READY, SET:

Grab the EZ-curl bar with an overhand, medium-width grip. Lie on a decline bench, hooking your feet under the pads. Hold the bar straight up over your chin—your upper arms should be nearly perpendicular to the floor.

GO:

Without moving your upper arms, slowly bend your elbows to lower the bar until it's just behind your head.

Pause, then slowly lift the bar back to the starting position. Repeat.

PERFORMANCE TIPS

■ As with any triceps exercise, keep your upper arms in one position throughout the exercise.

■ You can also try this exercise with dumbbells, using a neutral grip (palms facing each other).

Reverse Curl

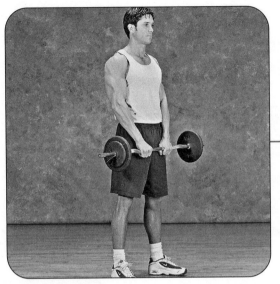

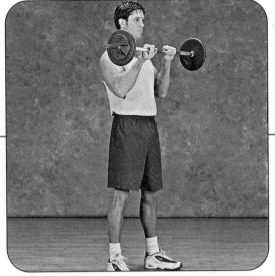

READY, SET:

Grab the EZ-curl bar with a medium-width, overhand grip. Hold the bar in front of your thighs, at arm's length, with your upper arms pressed against your sides, your shoulders back, your feet shoulder-width apart, and your knees slightly bent.

GO:

Without moving your upper arms, slowly bend your elbows to lift the bar as high as you can.

Pause, then slowly lower the bar back to the starting position. Repeat.

PERFORMANCE TIPS

■ When you perform this exercise slowly, keeping your upper arms pressed against your sides, you'll really feel it in your forearm-extensor muscles—the ones on top of your forearm in this movement. That's because those are the weakest muscles in your arms. But rest assured, you're also working your brachialis and brachioradialis, which add considerable size to your arms.

■ You can also do a reverse preacher curl in this routine. In that case, do it first, and then do a standard (underhand) biceps curl with the EZ-curl bar as your second biceps exercise.

■ Another variation is to do this using a low cable. Your arms will get more work on the lowering portion of the exercise, although you'll probably get more overall benefit doing this exercise with free weights.

Cable Pushdown

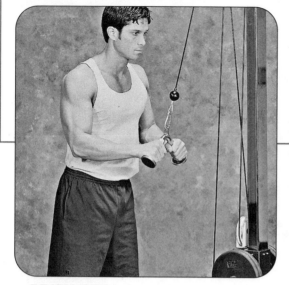
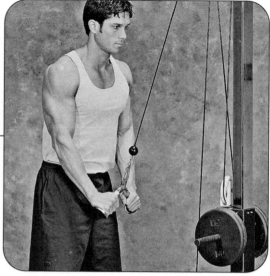

READY, SET:

Attach a V bar to the high cable pulley. Grab the bar with a medium-width, overhand grip. Stand in an athletic posture—feet shoulder-width apart, knees slightly bent. Press your upper arms against your sides. Lower the bar until your forearms are parallel to the floor and your elbows are bent 90 degrees.

GO:

Slowly push the bar down until your arms are straight and you feel the squeeze in your triceps.

Pause, then slowly return to the starting position. Repeat.

PERFORMANCE TIPS

■ This is one of the most popular exercises in the gym—and one that's almost never performed correctly. Almost everyone tries to add extra range of motion by starting with the bar up around chin level. That makes this a completely different exercise, engaging chest, back, and shoulder muscles. To isolate the triceps, start with your elbows bent 90 degrees.

■ Another common mistake is to start with your body bent at the waist, as if you were working a jackhammer. That engages the chest and shoulder muscles along with the triceps.

■ You can, though, turn this into a nice auxiliary abdominal exercise by keeping your midsection muscles contracted throughout the movement. It doesn't take anything away from the triceps to do this, as long as you keep your torso upright.

Standing High-Cable Curl

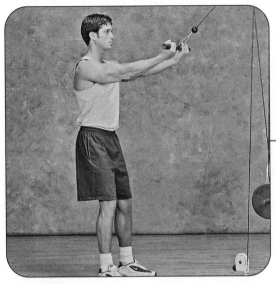 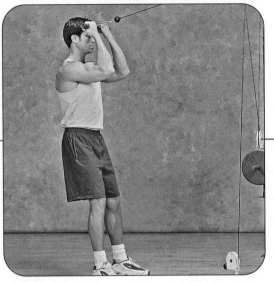

READY, SET:

Attach a straight bar to the high cable pulley. Grab the bar with a narrow, underhand grip, with your hands about 6 inches apart. Stand in an athletic posture—feet shoulder-width apart, knees slightly bent. Move back far enough that your arms are fully extended and parallel to the floor.

GO:

Without moving your upper arms, slowly bend your elbows to pull the bar toward your forehead. Pause to feel the squeeze in your biceps.

Slowly straighten your arms to return back to the starting position, and repeat.

PERFORMANCE TIPS

■ Keep your body in one position throughout the exercise; your elbows should be your only moving parts.

■ Toward the end of your set, you'll probably feel yourself rising up on your toes. Try to keep your heels flat on the floor.

Cable Reverse Pushdown

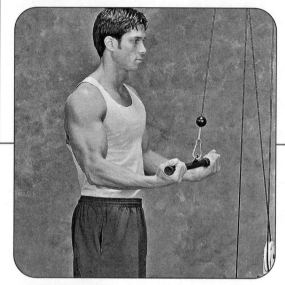 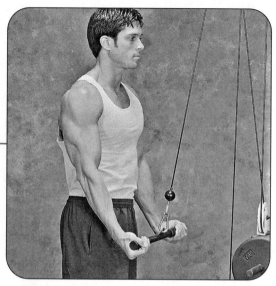

READY, SET:

Attach a straight bar to the high cable pulley. Grab the bar with an underhand grip, with your hands 12 to 18 inches apart. Stand in an athletic posture—feet shoulder-width apart, knees slightly bent. Press your upper arms against your sides. Lower the bar until your forearms are parallel to the floor and your elbows are bent 90 degrees.

GO:

Without moving your upper arms, slowly pull the bar down until your arms are straight and you feel the squeeze in your triceps.

Pause, then slowly return to the starting position. Repeat.

PERFORMANCE TIPS

- All the rules of triceps exercises apply here: Keep your body upright and your upper arms pressed against your sides.

- You'll feel an intense contraction in your triceps on this exercise, which will probably come as a shock at first and may even make you quit your sets before you do all your repetitions. Decrease the weight if you have to, but try to finish all your reps. You'll get used to the sharp contractions and be very pleased with the results you see.

- A good variation is to try this with one arm at a time, using a stirrup handle.

BODY BY YOU

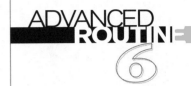

No weights? No problem. You're just a big dumbbell. This isn't an insult—it means that your own body is heavy enough to give your arms the resistance they need to get bigger and stronger.

All you need is a pair of parallel bars suitable for dips and a single bar on which you can do chinups. You can find these on any playground. You can also buy a chinup/dip station at any exercise-equipment store to keep in your home. Or you can do these exercises in a gym, if you're not in the mood to use that fully stocked weight room. Once you're proficient at chinups and dips, they could become an indispensable part of your arm workouts.

Do one to three sets of as many repetitions as you can, once or twice a week. Continue for as long as you keep increasing the total number of repetitions you can do from one workout to the next. Since these are maximum-effort exercises, you probably want to rest for at least 2 minutes between sets.

BODY-BY-YOU TRAINING LOG

Body-by-You Exercises	WEEK 1		WEEK 2		WEEK 3		WEEK 4	
	Workout 1	Workout 2	Workout 1	Workout 2	Workout 1	Workout 2	Workout 1	Workout 2
Chinup								
Dip								

Chinup

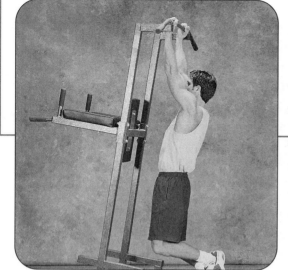

READY, SET:

Grab a chinup bar with an underhand grip, placing your hands a comfortable distance apart (probably less closer shoulder-width). Hang at arm's length with your feet crossed behind you.

GO:

Slowly bend your elbows and pull yourself up until your chin is above the bar.

Pause, then slowly lower yourself until your arms are straight again. Repeat.

PERFORMANCE TIPS

■ Keep your body still and straight; your shoulders and elbows should be your only moving parts.

■ Few guys can do high-repetition sets of chinups. You probably want to start with a near-maximum set—four, three, however many reps you can do. Then, try to do two more sets of nearly as many repetitions. In subsequent workouts, try to add one rep to each set until you can do multiple sets of six or more chinups.

■ The closer together you place your hands, the more you feel the exercise in your arms. And the farther apart you place them, the more you feel it in your back muscles. If you want to build your back, you're probably better off doing pullups, which is the same exercise using an overhand grip. You'll also want to place your hands farther than shoulder-width apart. Finally, you'll want to buy the next book in the *Men's Health* Peak Conditioning Guides series, *Essential Chest and Shoulders*.

Dip

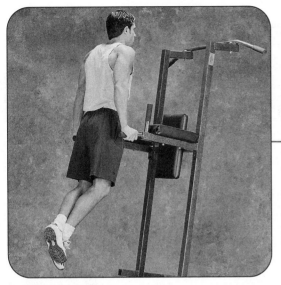 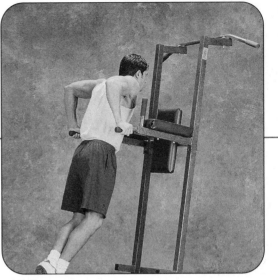

READY, SET:

Jump up on a pair of parallel bars and balance yourself with your arms fully straightened and your palms facing in. Keep your body as straight as possible, with your knees slightly bent and your feet crossed behind you.

GO:

Slowly bend your elbows and lower yourself until your upper arms are parallel to the floor.

Slowly push yourself back up to the starting position until your arms are straight again, and repeat.

PERFORMANCE TIPS

- Keep your body still and straight; your shoulders and elbows should be your only moving parts.

- You'll probably find that you can build up to sets of 10 or more dips more quickly than you can build up to sets of five or more chinups. To keep the repetitions equal between the two exercises—and thus work your biceps and triceps with equal intensity—you can wear a weighted belt when you do dips. Most gyms have a leather belt with a chain hanging down in front, to which you can attach a weight plate or dumbbell.

- The more upright your body, the more you work your triceps. And the more you lean forward, the more your dips emphasize your chest. But one aspect of the exercise that's universal is range of motion: Don't lower your body past the finishing position shown here. That can be way too tough on your shoulder joints.

CHAPTER FOURTEEN

ESSENTIAL LONG-RANGE PLAN

Weight training is a lifelong science project. The longer you train, the more you learn about what motivates you, what stimulates your muscles to grow, what combination of food and exercise gives you the most muscle with the least fat, what circumstances create the best training environment.

In other words, you become your own sports psychologist, exercise physiologist, nutritionist, and personal trainer. You'll do best in all those roles if you use a system called periodization, in which you create a plan outlining the workout changes you will make throughout a year or season.

Here's how you could structure that plan. Remember that after each training phase you should take a short break—anything from a couple of days to a week, depending on what you feel your body needs and how holidays and vacations fall in the calendar.

JANUARY:
MUSCLE ENDURANCE

Even the most dedicated exerciser feels a little bloated and soft after the Thanksgiving-to–New Year's pie-eating season. So when you hit the gym on January 2, do a single set of 12 to 15 repetitions of a dozen or so exercises. As the month progresses, work up to two and then three sets. Perform your workouts in a circuit fashion—that is, do one set of every exercise before doing a second set of any of them.

MUSCLE SIZE

Decrease your repetitions to 8 to 12 per set. Shift from circuits to straight sets—that is, do all your sets of a given exercise before moving on to the next exercise.

MARCH:
MUSCLE SIZE AND STRENGTH

Further decrease your repetitions to 6 to 10 per set.

APRIL:
MUSCLE STRENGTH

Decrease your repetitions to three to six per set, and increase your sets to as many as five for your most important exercises (bench press, squat, and bent-over row).

MAY:
VANITY

Your body probably feels pretty beaten up at this point from the hard work of building strength, so step back a little and focus on the muscle groups you most want to improve. Train those muscle groups first in your workouts, and increase repetitions to 8 to 12 per set.

JUNE:
GET CUT FOR SUMMER

Start with abdominal exercises, and increase repetitions once again to 10 to 15 per set. Add high-intensity techniques like supersets, drop sets (multiple sets of a single exercise without rest, decreasing the weight each set), and, if you're really serious about getting lean, "cardioresistance" workouts in which you do a set of a weight-lifting exercise followed by 2 to 3 minutes of a cardiovascular exercise.

JULY AND AUGUST:
ENJOY YOUR SUMMER

Now that you've built your body, shift to more flexible workouts. Work out when it's convenient, to maintain your muscle tone and most of your size. But also take every opportunity to get outside for a hike, swim, bike ride, or basketball game. You don't want your workouts to leave you so tired that you pass up chances to play.

SEPTEMBER:
BACK TO BASICS

Return to more formal, structured workouts, focusing on regaining your form on the most important exercises. Do 1 to 2 weeks' worth of workouts geared to regaining muscle endurance (12 to 15 repetitions per set), and spend the rest of the month on basic muscle building (8 to 12 repetitions).

OCTOBER:
MUSCLE SIZE AND STRENGTH

Perform 6 to 10 repetitions per set, using more weight each week.

NOVEMBER:
MUSCLE STRENGTH

Try to duplicate what you did in May, with heavier weights. If you can improve on all the weights you used at the end of May by 5 to 10 percent, you're doing things right.

PUMP UP FOR THE HOLIDAYS

There's a lot of stress around holiday time, so you don't want to add extremely stressful workouts to your physical and emotional burdens. Instead, pick the workouts that make you feel the best. These will probably be those that make your muscles feel the most pumped, or engorged with blood. The idea is to use your workouts to relieve stress, to make you feel better about yourself.

Take a week or two off from exercise so you can visit family and friends and indulge in all the holiday traditions. Your body needs breaks like this, so a week or two without exercise actually furthers the cause of your fitness. Don't feel that you're negating everything you worked so hard to develop throughout the year.

But make sure you don't abandon your workouts altogether—you need some exercise to maintain a jovial holiday mood and to counteract the excesses of the season. If your body does go visibly downhill during the holiday season, there's always January to get it back again.

INDEX

Underscored page references indicate boxed text.
Boldface references indicate photographs.